PRAKRITI &
PULSE

The two Mysteries of Ayurveda

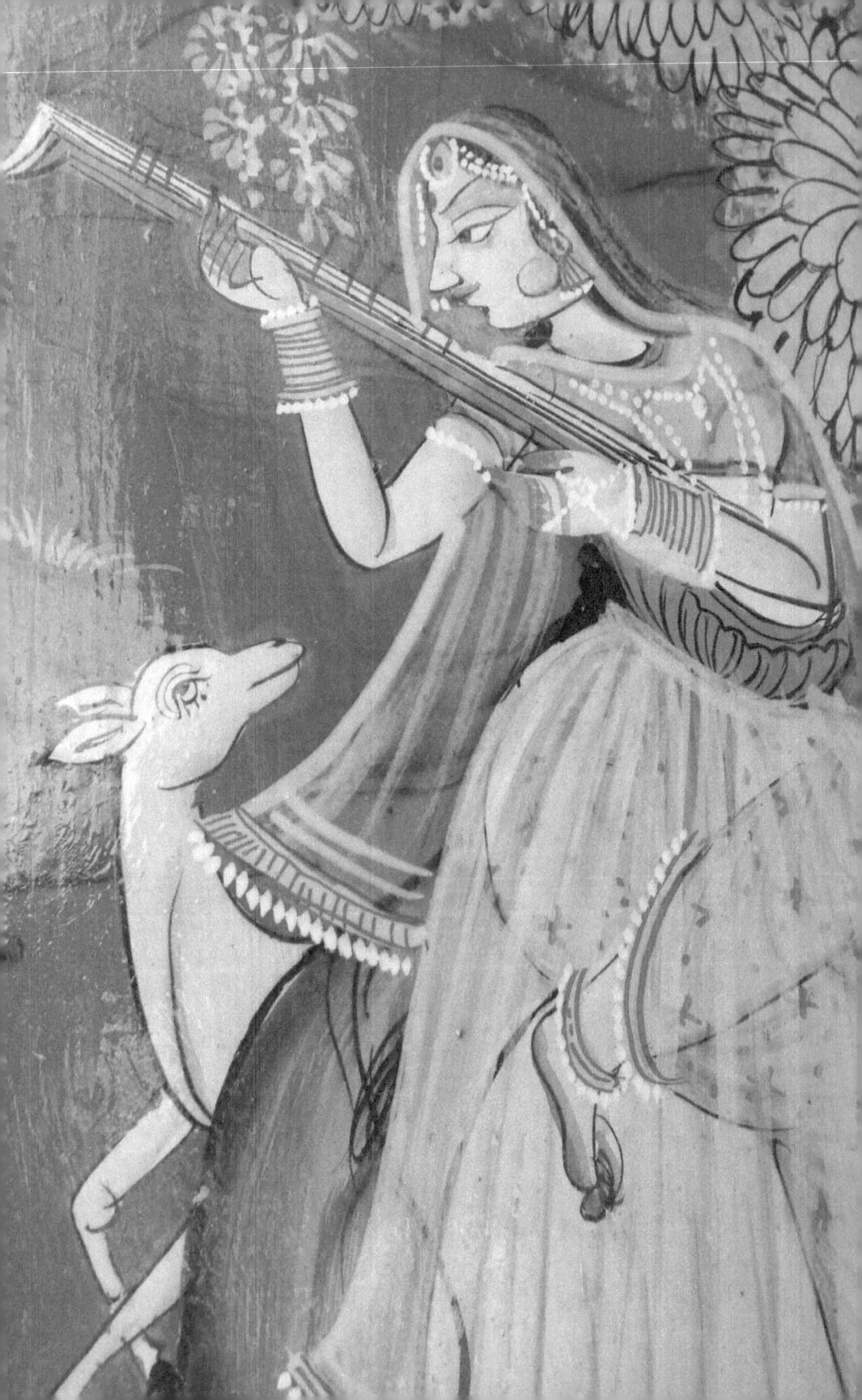

Dr. Vinod Verma

PRAKRITI & PULSE

The two Mysteries of Ayurveda

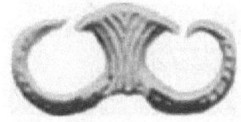

Gayatri Books International

The information provided in this book is not intended to replace the services of a physician. Diagnostic techniques and suggestions for a healthy way of living provided in this book are for the purpose of self-help and education. The author and the publisher are in no way responsible for any medical claims regarding the material presented in this book. For using methods and remedies provided in this book at commercial level requires the prior permission from the author. For more information, write to the author directly at ayurvedavv@yahoo.com

Translation rights are with the author. Write to the author directly at ayurvedavv@yahoo.com or ayurvedavv@gmail.com for translation rights.

Visit Dr. Vinod Verma at www.ayurvedavv.com and www.drvinodverma.com to find out about her seminars, lectures and consultations, etc. Information is also provided at the back pages of the book.

Consultant: Mohit Joshi
Design and photographs by the author
 ISBN: 978-1499327922
         1499327927

Dedicated to Khushwant Singh, a great writer of all times, a superb human being and a warm hearted friend who left us on 20 March 2014 at the age of 99

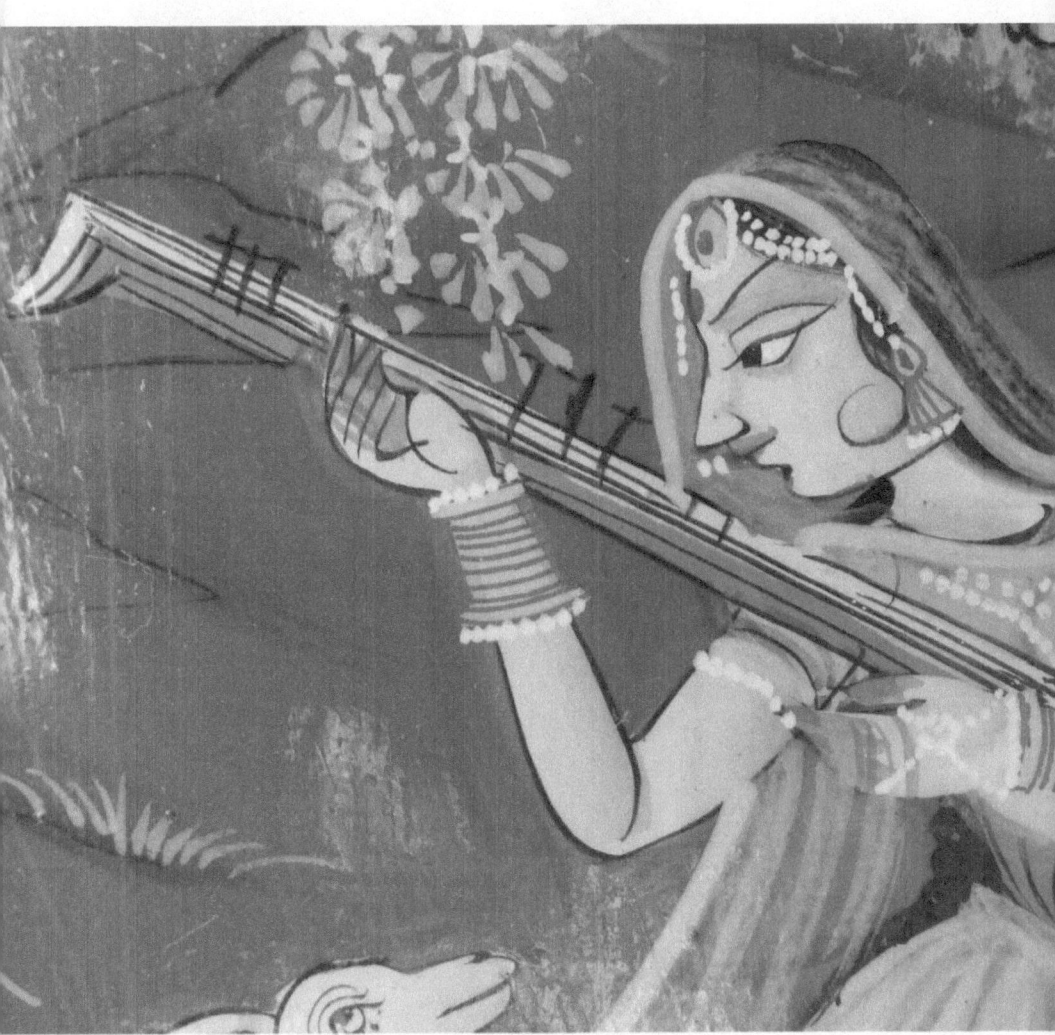

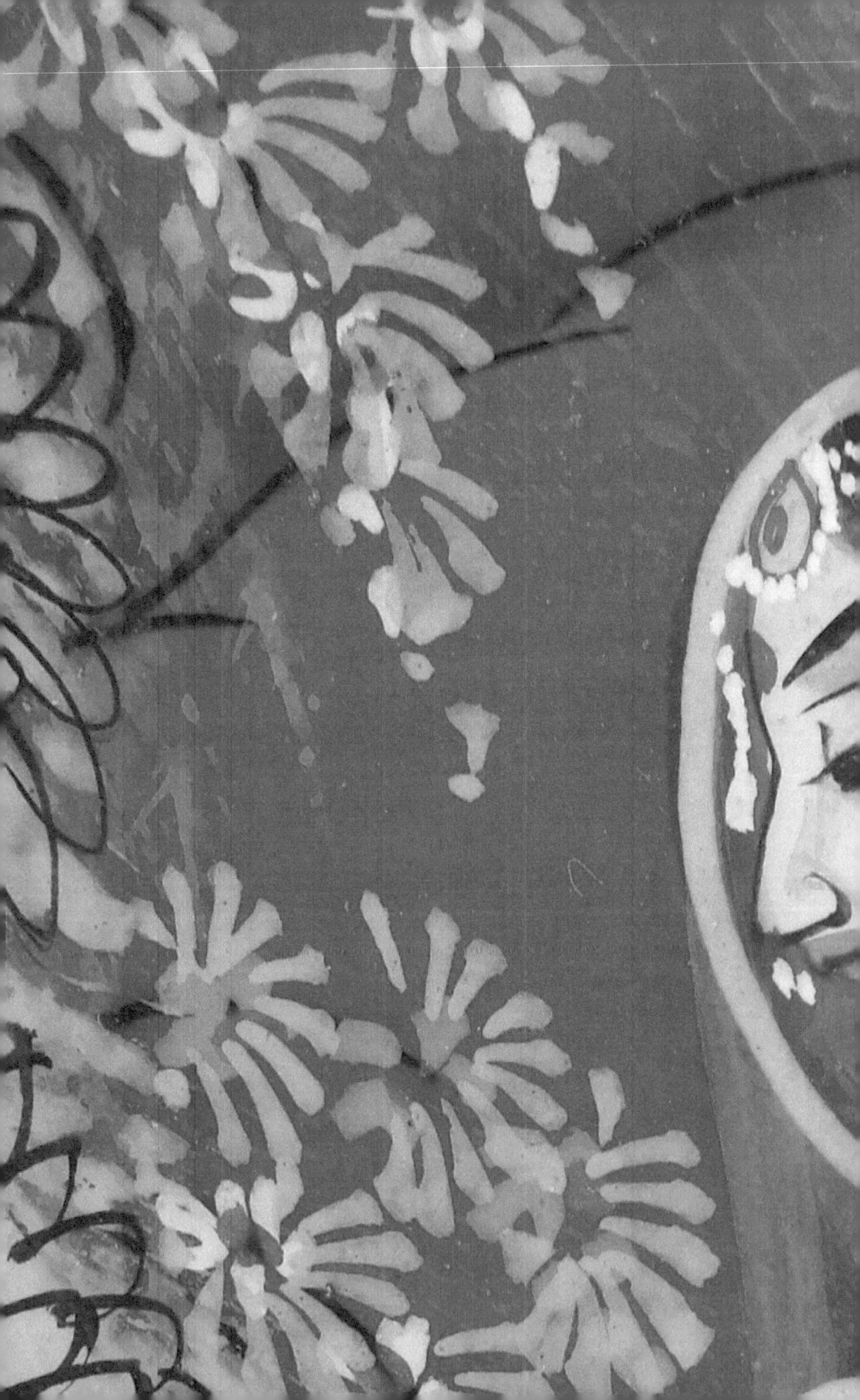

Preface

I have been writing books on Ayurveda and also have been teaching for nearly three decades. My experience reveals that two very important aspects of Ayurveda, which make it fascinating for the Westerners, are: Prakriti– the individual constitution and Nadi Pariksha– the pulse examination for diagnosis. Prakriti is not only the fundamental human constitution at physiological level, but also denotes the basic personality of an individual. People find it fascinating and are many times mystified in my classes when I tell them just by looking at them about their basic likes and dislikes, as well as their fundamental behavioural patterns. The pulse examination by an Ayurvedic physician reveals prakriti as well as the state of a person's health. There is again a surprise element in it from the point of view of an average westerner. In fact, these two aspects, which are the fundamental wisdom of Ayurveda in India, are rather mystified in the West. When people call me for a private session in Europe, they want to make sure beforehand that these two will be a part of the session, as they find them very fascinating. Both these methods reveal something about a human being without undergoing complicated tests with sophisticated machines. Nevertheless, they are not methods of healing but of diagnose. Therefore, I think it is more the mystical element in both these methods that attracts people.

Prakriti: the individual identity, diagnosis and prevention

The knowledge of Prakriti is not only extremely important for health, healing and prescription of the remedies in Ayurveda, but is also the fundamental basis of human psychology. The most important aspect of prakriti is that it provides an individual identity, which forms the basis for a personal space and freedom within his/her social framework. One has to learn to accept that some of us are slower than the others and are more patient and tolerant. On the contrary, there are others who get easily angry. There are some who are so quick to decide whereas there are others who find hard to take a decision. Once we attribute the fundamental individual variations to nature, we learn to accept others as they are.

Wisdom about prakriti helps to accept the human variations and is a key to enhance understanding at familial and social levels. It can be used to enhance work efficiency, as well as harmony at work place.

Prakriti ascertains your identity and individuality, though at a very basic level. Due to the prevalence of mechanistic view of life for the last two hundred years, all human beings are treated like machines and at the same level. Parents tell their children: Why cannot you be like your brother (or sister)? Couples tell each other: Why cannot you get dressed quickly like I do? A friend or someone in a group may be condemned for not deciding quickly or sleeping too much. Another may be criticized for eating too much

8

or too little. With the concept of prakriti that ascertains natural variation in individuals, people get some breathing space for being and accepting what they are.

Prakriti is the fundamental human identity and any diversion from this state is termed as vikriti (unnatural, a state of vitiation). This diversion helps us to diagnose the state of health of a person. Thus, the diversion from the state of health or one's natural state of being indicates that a person is heading towards the state of being unwell. Ayurvedic wisdom provides us the knowledge which enables us to restore back to the state of perfection (prakriti) from the state that takes us towards illness (vikriti). Illness or disorder mostly is born from a constant state of vikriti or chronic vikriti. Thus, the knowledge about prakriti and the wisdom to maintain it is a great step in preventive medicine.

Pulse: the diagnosis and the music of life

Pulse is the music of life in our body. It helps us not only to diagnose our state of health but also enhances the sensitivity towards our own body. We discover that there is an ever-changing rhythm within us that gets affected with the change in our inner and outer environment. Learning about the pulse paves way for understanding of oneself and to de-mechanise the way of living. It also specifically helps those of you who lead very mind-oriented lives and are indifferent to the throbbing and pulsating 'ground reality'. Knowledge of pulse and its ever-changing rhythm help provide us the consciousness of the living element within us, thus leading an understanding of our system as an ever changing whole. Remember that pulse is the sign of life throbbing in us; it is the warmth, vivacity and energy. It gives us the consciousness of our dynamic body and appreciation for being alive. Wisdom and experience of pulse examination is a journey in profound layers of our existence. Learning about pulse examination, its scope and its limitations will help people as well as therapists to discover the subtle aspects of human existence.

Since there is a growing number of Ayurvedic therapists in the West and more and more people are using Ayurvedic healing methods the world over, it is important to have the fundamental literature available in foreign languages. At the moment, the important literature is in Sanskrit and Hindi and besides that, it is scattered all over in different bodies of literature. The therapists in India and abroad do not have an access to comprehensive and precise literature on the subject. Besides that, people who would like to use Ayurvedic methods of health and healing should have literature available to inform them properly in a scientific manner before they subject themselves to Ayurvedic therapies.

The vibrant cosmos and dynamic body

Everything in the cosmos is changing from one state to another constantly. Cosmos is a dynamic whole and there is a fundamental unity in all what exists. In the modern world, the human beings, especially the ones residing in the metros, do not understand this dynamism of nature and of their own bodies. That is why they get numerous health problems related to both body and mind. There are many spiritual schools in the cities the world over but generally they mystify the human reality and do not explain scientifically. The knowledge and the practical aspects of these two ancient Ayurvedic practices will help people understand scientifically about the dynamic and vibrant aspect of our existence. This wisdom will not only help you to understand your body and the nature of the cosmos, but also the profound aspects of human psyche. The mental problems and social frictions generally have their roots in not comprehending the variability of human mind. It is the lack of understanding that every second the cosmos changes and it is no more the same as it was a second earlier.

Thus, the practical wisdom provided in this book will not only help you comprehend your own body and mind, but also will lead you to a better understanding of life at familial, social and spiritual level. First we understand the vibrant aspect of our own body, then of our surroundings and finally we begin to see the dynamic cosmos we inhabit.

Practical wisdom

One cannot attain the knowledge about prakriti and pulse exclusively by reading books or attending a week-end seminar. It takes me 300 hours of teaching with my students to make them confident in prakriti.

Prakriti and Pulse

After doing practical exercises in the class, we go to streets, gardens and cafés for practice. With all this, students reach at a level that observation becomes compulsive and they observe prakriti automatically.

The purpose of this book is to teach you practical wisdom of both pulse and prakriti. Therefore, the book has also the practical exercises. It is impossible to learn these themes fast and put them in practice. They are learnt both by practice and experience.

Ayurveda is the mother medicine of all the medicines of the world and is 5000 years old. Ayurvedic sages have contributed to it through experimentations and experience through ages and have enriched this wisdom. Therefore, it is suggested that the therapist using this book should learn with patience and endeavour before putting them to practice. The book provides commonsensical wisdom of day-to-day life which can help to know oneself better, as well to understand others better. For readers with no background of Ayurveda, I have given a concise introduction along with references.

Vinod Verma
www.ayurvedavv.com
ayurvedavv@yahoo.com   ayurvedavv@gmail.com

Contents

Part II
Nadi Priksha: The Pulse Diagnose

Introduction to Ayurveda

"Ayurveda is that which deals with good-bad, happy-unhappy [aspects of] life, promoters and non-promoters [of life] and their nature and measurements".*

This precise and pithy definition of Ayurveda, given by the sage himself 2600 years ago describes all. This definition also shows you the scientific approach of Charaka as he tells us that fundamental is to know the nature and measurements of all that which promotes and diminish life, all that which is good or bad for our existence, all that which brings us comfort and balance or contrary to it. In Sanskrit, there are two words: sukh and dukh, which are usually translated as happiness and unhappiness*. But in reality sukh is a satisfied and balanced state of mind and dukh denotes frustration, longing and an imbalanced state of mind. Once we know the nature and measurements of these factors, we can work precisely to promote life along with human happiness and well being. These factors include all aspects of existence: concrete, material, subtle and abstract.

---

* *Charaka Samhita,* Sutrasthana, I, 41
* For details, please see my article in Ayurveda Sutra on Sukha, Volume I, issue 10.

Prakriti and Pulse

The basic wisdom of yoga and Ayurveda is thousands of years old but their popularity the world over during the last two decade indicates that this wisdom is eternal. Only eternal wisdom can provide eternal solutions. Eternal wisdom is beyond space and time and it does not belong to any country but is the world heritage.

Many people, both home and abroad, have this misconception that Ayurveda is exclusively a medical system. Ayurveda is a Veda of life and ailments also belong to life. Life has an order and a system. Temporary disorders and ailments are a part of life. Thus, the Veda of life, helps us to understand what life is, how to organise and manage our lives, how to prevent ailments and in case of ailments, how to get back to health. Ayurveda teaches us to live our lives with optimum level of energy for the maximum length of time. Longevity, sexuality and rejuvenation are as much a part of Ayurveda as treating ailments. The Ayurvedic advices on lifestyle for maintaining good health, enhancing energy, preventing ailments and treating minor ailments are integrated in ceremonious tradition of India and in its food culture. The traditional Indian kitchen is set up in such a way that it is also a little apothecary. This culture is nearly lost in the Indian metros and most young people do not even recognize different spices what to talk of preparing some home remedies. The city dwellers generally buy readymade masalas (spice mixtures) and thus children do not grow up learning the basic wisdom of Ayurvedic food culture and its simple healing methods.

The fundamental basis of Ayurveda

The principles of Ayurveda are based on cosmic unity. In this cosmos, everything is interconnected and interdependent. Causative factor of the basic cosmic unity is the common constituent of all what exists. The dynamic, ever changing cosmos constituted of the five fundamental elements (ether or space, air, fire, water and earth) has two principal divisions according to Ayurveda: *jadda* and *chetana*. *Jadda* are all the non-livings whereas *chetana* are those with soul and have their independent functional system. In *chetana,* the five elements take the form of three doshas or three principal energies – vata, pitta and kapha. The three doshas perform all the physical and mental functions of the body. It is important to understand that jadda or so called non-living is also dynamic and changes with time. Rivers change their courses, stones change their shapes, caves are formed and the quality of the earth change with time.

The dynamic body and the three doshas

Vata is constituted from elements ether and air and its functions are related to these two elements. Ether or space is omnipresent and air is mobile. The functions related to movements as well as to space are performed by vata.

17

Vata is responsible for entire body movements, blood circulation, respiration, excretion, speech, sensations, touch, hearing, feelings like fear, anxiety, grief, enthusiasm etc., natural urges, formation of foetus, sexual act and retention.

Fire constitutes pitta energy of the body and thus pitta is body's fire or *agni*. When we use the word agni in Ayurveda, it pertains to everything related to digestion and assimilation. Agni in Ayurvedic terminology is a part of pitta but as you see pitta has also some other functions.

Pitta is responsible for vision, hunger, thirst, heat regulation, softness, lustre, cheerfulness, intellect and sexual vigour.

Kapha forms the solid part of the body and is responsible for the formation of new cells. Also when we are adult, our body constantly needs new cells. We need various secretions in the body. The inner lining of the uterus is made of endothelial cells and these are constantly renewed.

Kapha constitutes all the solid structure of the body and is responsible for binding different body organs together. It gives rise to firmness and heaviness to the body and is responsible for sexual potency, strength, forbearance and restraint.

Both body and cosmos are dynamic and they have the same fundamental constituents- the five elements. Just as we need the equilibrium of five elements in the cosmos for an order and harmony in the cosmic system, similarly, for good health, we need a balance of these elements, which constitute our body in the form of three energies. To imagine five elements in the body in the form of vata, pitta and kapha may sound abstract. It is easier to comprehend the system of three energies in the body and their equilibrium if we first understand how five elements maintain the cosmic equilibrium and what happens when this equilibrium is disturbed.

Imagine a calm day when it is neither too hot nor too cold. The wind is blowing mildly and there is a perfect ratio of humidity in the air. Everything seems serene and calm and you feel good in this kind of atmosphere. Imagine another day with very fast winds blowing. The wind can uproot trees or destroy other things. If the trees fall in a river, there is a danger of flood. First of all, the element wind was not in equilibrium. It disturbed the element earth and uprooted the trees. The trees were no more there where they should have been and they were there where they should not be. Thus, the fast winds also disturb the element space. In case of flood, the element water is also disturbed as it enters into the fields and destroys the crops. Once again, the element earth is disturbed. Thus we see that when one of the elements in nature does not function properly, the whole system is disturbed. Similarly, for good health, the three energies or dosha of the body, made from five elements, should perform their functions in harmony with each other. If one of the energies is disturbed, we step into a state of imbalance and ill health.

We can also take other examples from nature. When the summer is too hot or it does not rain and there is drought, or there are accidents with the life-giving fire or there are floods or earthquakes, there is destruction. Similarly, when we do not maintain the equilibrium of the five elements in our system, there are disturbances and ill health. In other words, our system is built the same way as nature. If we go against nature, eat too much or too little or too frequently or do not sleep during the night or sleep during the day and do not care to go to the toilet on time, and so on, our system is disturbed with these anti-natural acts.

These energies are constantly being used and are replenished through breathing and our food. Through breathing we get the cosmic energy or prana shakti. The air we breathe in does not only have oxygen to pump our heart, it has the light and warmth of the sun during the day, tender energy of the night and special fragrance of each season. Thus, with breathing we inhale all the five elements of the cosmos in the form of subtle energy. Therefore, it is very important to breathe rightly and learn some basic pranayama practices. Pranayama is conscious and controlled breathing. In the polluted cities, we suffer from prana vikriti or vitiation. Our food provides us the five elements in the concrete form to rebuild the three vital energies.

Same principles apply to all the cosmos including the human body. Just like the balance of the five elements is essential in the cosmos and excessive wind, fire accidents, floods and earthquakes are destructive; similarly the three doshas should be balanced in the body for good health and harmony.

Prakriti

Each individual has a fundamental constitution or prakriti from birth and this denotes his or her basic appearance and fundamental behaviour. Thus, the physical and the mental aspects of human beings are interwoven and interdependent. Diversity in prakriti is due to the domination of one or more doshas.

Individual constitution or prakriti has seven major types and numerous subtypes.

1. Vata
2. Pitta
3. Kapha
4. Vata-pitta
5. Pitta kapha
6. Kapha vata
7. Samadosha (all doshas are balanced)

The numerous variations in each of the seven types of prakriti are due to the variation in the degree of dominance of a dosha, variable proportion of the two doshas in mixed prakriti and the difference in the fundamental physical and mental energy we bring with us due to our past karma at the time of birth.

Prakriti, Vikriti and ailments

Prakriti is influenced by external factors like place, weather, climate, time of the day, age, emotions and other special circumstances like travelling, etc. For good health and harmony, an individual has to make an effort to maintain his/her state of prakriti by following a lifestyle according to space and time (*desha* and *kala*). There is a description of *dinacharya* (the daily routine) and *ritucharaya* (the seasonal routine) in Ayurvedic texts. If we do not pay attention to diverse factors influencing us in this dynamic cosmos and mould our lifestyle according to the external factors, we can temporarily feel unwell or we come in the state of vikriti. For example, the windy weather can cause vata vikriti and you may feel stiffness in the body, get constipation, get dry throat or may feel restless. Hot weather can cause pitta vikriti and you may get excessive perspiration, body smell, abnormal hunger and thirst, rash, pimples and blisters. Cold and rainy weather can cause kapha vikriti and you may feel drowsy, get sweet taste in mouth, excessive salivation, nausea etc. Childhood is kapha, youth is pitta and the old age is vata in predominance.

All our life, we change from prakriti to vikriti and vice versa. It is a natural process and body re-establishes its harmony and reverts back to its natural state from vikriti. This change from vikriti to prakriti is quicker during youth when one has high vitality and immunity (ojas) and longer during childhood and old age. For a better understanding of the Ayurvedic principles it is very important to comprehend the dynamism of our body system and that of the cosmos.

PRAKRITI 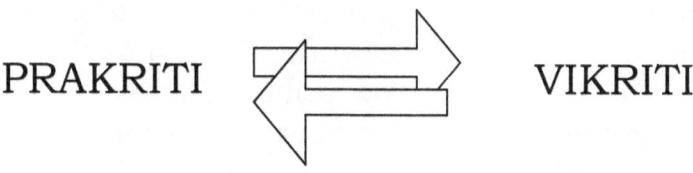 VIKRITI

If we leave the state of vikriti unattended and lead a lifestyle that further disturbs it, we become sick. If we further neglect it over a long period of time, we become prey to a serious ailment or an incurable disorder. For example, vata vikriti with symptoms of stiffness in the body gives rise to chronic body ache over a period of time and if still not properly attended to, one gets arthritis.

Daily Diagnose

For keeping in good health and for maintaining a state of well being, we have to make every effort to retain our state of prakriti. There are several external features and our excretions that help us to diagnose our state of health. Pulse is amongst the eight types of diagnoses described in Ayurveda. These are done from examination of stool, urine, tongue, voice, skin, eyes, general appearance and pulse.

It is the responsibility of an individual to keep the body in a good shape by observation and simple diagnostic analysis and take immediate action to revert back to the state of prakriti from vikriti.

Individual duty to maintain health is called svadharma. All the eight kinds of diagnosis help us to deduct our present state of health and provide guidance to take an appropriate action to maintain health. Excretions of the body reveal to us the inner state of the body. Yellow urine indicates too much heat in the body, dry and hard stool is the indicative of vata vikriti whereas a sticky stool and foamy urine indicate kapha vikriti.

Importance of pulse examination is that blood flows in each and every part of the body and any abnormality in any part of the body is indicated in its pulsation. But it is long and hard to learn this subtle method of diagnose. Like learning music, it needs constant practice and experience.

The three states of mind

Before we proceed further to understand the concept health, it is important to understand that besides three doshas, our state of mind influences our health. According to Ayurveda, mind has three major characteristics qualities– sattva, rajas and tamas. The rajas quality of mind includes thinking, planning and taking decisions. The tamas quality is that which hinders motion (like state of sleep, fatigue or laziness) and restricts the expansion of mind (e.g. emotions like greed, anger, jealousy, etc.). The sattva quality of mind includes equilibrium, goodness, truth, compassion, stillness and peace. Sattva helps balance rajas and tamas, which predominate our modern life. Lack of sattva not only influences the equilibrium of the doshas but also causes mental

24

ailments. Thus, for maintaining good health and longevity, a six dimensional equilibrium is essential as the three dimensions at two levels mutually influence each other.

Our state of mind influences our principal energies (vata, pitta and kapha), which are responsible for the physical and mental functions of the body. For example, if we are worried or are over-worked or have excessive mental stress, we are in rajas state of mind. In this case, we get vata vikriti and suffer from symptoms like restlessness, disturbed sleep, constipation or stiffness in the body or some other symptoms of vata vikriti. Too much anger (tamas) influences pitta and one can suffer from pitta related disorders like stomach ailments. Depression (tamas) gives rise to kapha related disorders leading to obesity, nausea, excessive salivation, etc. State of imbalance of the three doshas also influences our state of mind. For example, if constipation or partial evacuation persists, it can give rise to sleep disorders or hectic mental state or nervous behaviour. Stomach problems, which are due to pitta disturbances, may enhance anger and irritation. Excessive sleep, which is a sign of kapha vikriti may give rise to depression.

Thus, it is important to understand that for keeping the basic equilibrium of the body, a six dimensional effort is required. It is not enough to balance the doshas to attain perfect health. Equally important is to maintain a mental equilibrium and attain a sense of satisfaction. Charaka lays a great emphasis on sattva for maintaining balance between rajas and tamas states of mind. Santosha or a state of contentment is one aspect of sattva and according to Charaka, asantosha or a state of discontentment is one of the principal causes of ailments.

The six dimensional equilibrium

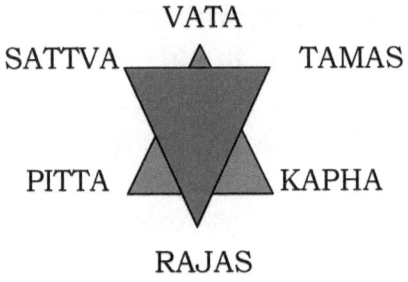

VATA

SATTVA   TAMAS

PITTA   KAPHA

RAJAS

Rasa in food

We replenish our three vital forces through breathing and nourishment. In our food, we have six different tastes- sweet, sour, salty, bitter, pungent and astringent. Our tongue indicates the taste just as our eyes see the colours. Each taste has an influence on the totality of our body as it brings two fundamental elements to our body to rebuild the three doshas. This total effect of a taste is called rasa in Ayurvedic pharmacology. We should balance our daily diet by making sure that we have no rasa in excess in our food and neither we leave out any. Rasa theory is the basis of Ayurvedic pharmacology and nutrition.

Appropriate physical activity

Ayurveda lays a great emphasis on appropriate physical activity— to do yogic exercise and asanas (posture) as well as take morning and evening walks. Sedentary lifestyle closes the energy channels of the body called the *srotas* and leads to numerous ailments like numbness in different parts of the body, arteriosclerosis, over-weight and weariness. However, an excessive physical activity or walking too much give rise to vata vikriti and should be avoided.

Three types of diseases

In the classical Ayurveda, diseases are three kinds:
  1. The first kind is born out of imbalance of doshas. They are mainly lifestyle ailments.
  2. The second category of disease is due to external attacks like virus, bacteria, poisons or accidents, etc.
  3. The third kind includes mental diseases and they originate from excessive rajas and tamas.

The three kinds of disease are inter-related as the first category can make one weak and vulnerable to the second and third category of diseases as well. Similarly, the second and third categories lead to imbalance of the doshas.

Three types of therapies

Rational, mental and spiritual are three kinds of therapies in Ayurveda and they should be applied

27

simultaneously. They are not exclusive of each other. Besides the drugs, rational therapy includes directions on lifestyle, nutrition, therapeutic yoga, diverse kinds of heat treatments, anointing, etc.

Mental and spiritual therapies along with the rational therapy are a very important part of the Ayurvedic therapeutics and in this regard, there is a great emphasis on sattva.

The great sage of Ayurveda, Charaka wrote 2600 years ago:

> **"Conceit, fear, anger, greed, ignorance, narcosis and confusion, troublesome actions taken under spell and other actions arisen from *rajas* and *tamas* are due to intellectual error (*pragyapradha*) and are the cause of diseases."**

> **"The persons having dominating *sattva* are endowed with memory, devotion, are grateful, learned, pure, courageous, skilful, resolute, fighting in battles with prowess, free from anxiety, having well directed and serious intellect and activities and are engaged in virtuous acts"**

Inner and outer purification

According to Ayurveda, the deposit of mala in the body causes ailments. There are all kinds of daily purification practices in Dincharya- the daily routine. There are simple things like drinking a glass of hot water in the morning upon getting up, going for a walk, doing yoga and ensuring proper evacuation two times a day, etc. The outer cleanliness and care of the body should be insured with cleaning the buccal cavity, ears, nasal passage, anal and vaginal openings, morning bath and oiling the body and so many other small and easy to do practices. Every six months, after the principal seasons, in the months of September and October, and March and April, the inner purification practices (panchakarma) are suggested. These practices are also integrated in our ceremonious practices as the nine days of partial fast during the navaratra.*

Rasayana

Rasayanas are the substances or groups of substances which have special properties and rasas in intensity. Rasayanas enhance the ojas (immunity and vitality) and rejuvenate body and mind. Ayurveda suggests a regular intake of rasayanas to enhance energy, longevity and to maintain youth and vigour. Ayurvedic spices are rasayanas. Garlic, ginger, cumin, fennel, pippali (Long pepper) are some examples. However, they should be taken in right combinations and doses to have the rejuvenating effect.

---

* For more details, please refer to my books: *Ayurveda: A Way of Life, Ayurveda for Inner Harmony: Nutrition, Sexual Energy and Healing, Programming Your Life with Ayurveda* and *Stress-free Work with Yoga and Ayurveda*. These books are available at www.amazon.com.

Prakriti and Pulse

To sum up, right breathing, appropriate body activities through exercise and yoga to open srotas or the energy channels, balanced nutrition with all the rasas, use of rasayanas, right evacuation, inner and outer purifications, sattvic mental state and *santosha* are some key factors for good health. For doing all this, you need to make an effort at the individual level. We have to make every effort to maintain our natural state of health- prakriti. Our prakriti is our first identity. We have to learn to diagnose any diversion from prakriti to vikriti or a state of being unwell. Ailments and disorders result due to chronic vikriti, which is caused due to a long state of neglect.

Part I

PRAKRITI:

The inner

human face

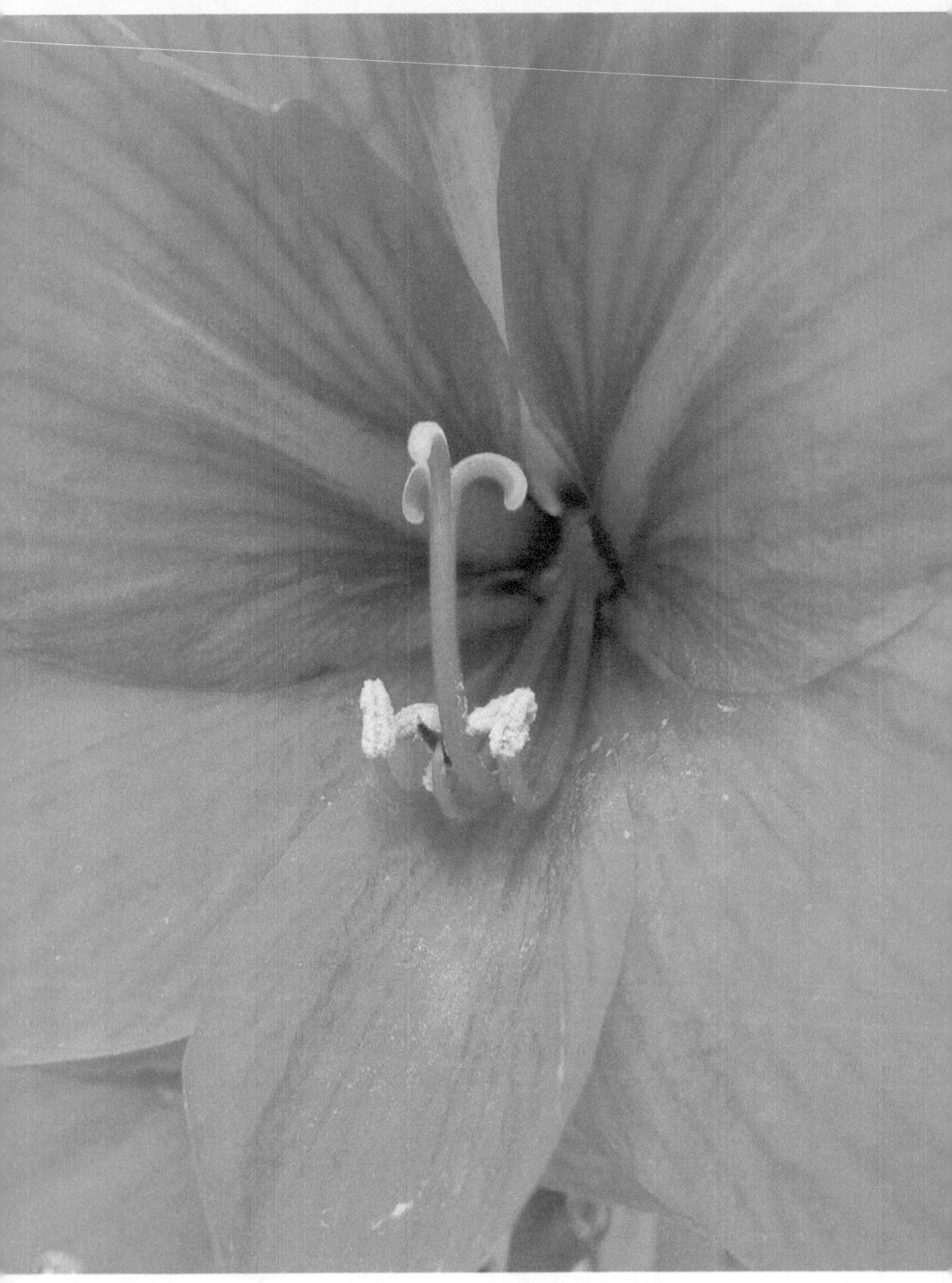

1

Prakriti–our Natural Being

The literal meaning of the word prakriti is nature. In the present context, prakriti is our fundamental nature and we are born with it. It can be called as *fundamental human constitution* but you should keep in mind that it also includes aptitudes, attitudes, basic talents and abilities as well. We are all born with these different basic traits. Just like we all look different outwardly though we all have two eyes, one nose, two ears, etc., similarly prakriti denotes our inner identity. As parents cannot decide about the looks of the baby they are going to have, similarly, they also cannot decide about the prakriti of the baby. Both, outward and inward appearances come naturally with the little being at birth.

Prakriti does not mean that an individual is condemned to be in a certain way or have some typical traiots of one sort. The freedom lies in ability to discern (buddhi) and ability to act (present karma called purushkara in Ayurveda). Our outward appearance, as well as prakriti is like a terrain. Wisdom lies in making an effort to work on ourselves and grow trees according to the nature of that terrain. This will yield the best of fruits. The other advice is to be satisfied with the fruits of one's own terrain and not compare it to the fruits of the other's terrain.

You see around you different variety of trees. They are all trees but they have different foliage, different flowers and fruits and in different seasons. Similarly variations in human being, both inwardly and outwardly are very natural. There is no value judgement attached to this natural variation.

Theoretical basis of prakriti

The word prakriti means *nature*. Prakriti also means the Cosmic Substance. According to the tradition of Samkhya, Yoga and Ayurveda, the phenomenal world begins when two principle energies come together- Purusha (Universal Energy) and Prakriti (Cosmic Substance). Prakriti has the substance but is lifeless whereas Purusha has life but cannot act as it has no vehicle to act. Prakriti has three characteristic qualities and they come in action only when Purusha puts life into Prakriti. These qualities or gunas are sattva, rajas and tamas.

The rajas is the quality of action and movement in the cosmos. Tamas is that quality which hinders motion as opposite to rajas. Rajas expands in space whereas tamas shrinks. The sattva quality denotes equilibrium and purity. In fact this quality balances rajas and tamas.

The Cosmic Substance or Prakriti is the inherent cosmic nature with its three characteristic qualities or gunas. In the phenomenon world, each individual

34

is an independent entity with its own system of mind and body. Though fundamentally, the body functions on the same principles as cosmos, but an individual has a sense of discretion and intellect and is responsible for his/her own deeds (karma). Time is eternal and cyclic and the results of the karma are carried further beyond one life span. The results of the karma also appear in one life span but the sum total that remains at the time of death is decisive for the conditions of birth and state of health during the next birth. This is a decisive factor for an individual's outer appearance as well as for inner face– the prakriti or the fundamental constitution.

The cosmic interaction is on the basis of cause and effect. We do good to someone and it comes back to us. We plant trees and nature will shower blessing on us. We cut trees or damage environment in another way, we have to pay back for it. The cosmic interaction is programmed and karma and its accountability work by itself. There is no God or similar power which is responsible for our good or bad health, beauty, wealth or misery. It is all an individual's own doing and each one of us are reaping our own harvest.

At the time of birth, we bring a suitcase full of the former karma with us. Along with other things like in the kind of family we are born, it also determines our state of health, our fundamental personality traits, our inherent nature and our basic constitution. The results of the past karma appear in the form of sanskara in the present life. Sanskara is our inherent nature and aptitudes. Sanskara is, in a way the, extension of the memory of the past life or lives that appear in the form of our inherent interests, gifts, aptitudes, kindness, violence or any number of other positive or negative traits. Thus, prakriti or the fundamental constitution, like many other things is pre-determined. We are born with certain fundamental constitution or prakriti, just like we are born with certain physical features that makes our appearance. Just like our appearance stays with us all our lives, similarly, our prakriti, as our inner being, remains the same throughout our lives.

2
Prakriti Determination

First step to learn about prakriti determination is to learn about the characteristics of each type of prakriti in order to understand the basic human variations in physical reactions and fundamental personality traits.

Physical features and personality traits of individuals with vata prakriti

1. Intolerant to cold and shiver easily
2. Agile
3. Quick and unrestricted in their movements
4. Swift in actions
5. Dry skin
6. Smoky eyes and rather dull complexion
7. Coarse hair and nails
8. Prominent blood vessels
9. Quick to worry, get easily

fearful and in general rapid in the display of emotions
10.   Get easily irritated

Physical features and personality traits of individuals with pitta prakriti

1. Intolerant to heat
2. Have usually a hot face
3. Delicate organs
4. Tendency to have moles, freckles and pimples
5. Lustrous complexion and reddish eyes
6. Excessive hunger and thirst
7. Tendency to have hair fall
8. Body odour
9. Intolerance and lack of endurance
10.   Get easily angry specially when hungry

Physical features and personality traits of individuals with kapha prakriti

1. Slow in activities and speech
2. Stable movements
3. Well united and strong ligaments
4. Clear eyes, face and complexion
5. Little hunger, thirst or perspiration
6. Disorderly
7. Delayed initiation
8. Slow to take decisions
9. Patient and tolerant
10.   Generally satisfied

Principal observations for prakriti determination

I have given below the three basic dimensions for observing a human being in order to identify his or her prakriti. In each case, many different points should be observed. It is quite possible that you may get confused with some of the observations. But observing other related aspects will solve this problem.

1. External appearance

The most basic observation for determining prakriti as well as to know the state of your health is your outward appearance, like eyes, complexion, nature of the skin, quantity and quality of the hair, body structure and other features of an individual's appearance.

2. Physical reactions

The second step to determine prakriti is to observe the physical reactions of people to various life situations. For example to note the physical reactions of people to a stress situation, a shocking news, a good news, an exciting news, an emergency, and so on. When under stress or in a bad situation, some may have frequent stool or urination, the others may get constipation, there are still others who may vomit. Some may just sleep or remain dumbfounded. On long-term stress situations like at work, various persons display diverse reactions. Some may get stomach problems or other ailments related to digestive system. There are others, who may get different kinds of aches. Another type of persons may start sleeping too much and also get depressed.

3. Behaviour

The way people walk, talk, climb up stairs, enter into a room, answer their doorbells or telephones reveal their prakriti. I have talked above about the physical reactions various people have in different life situations. In this category, notice the behavioural aspect of their reactions. When something goes wrong, people react differently. Does a person gets angry or keeps patience? While narrating something, various persons have different ways. Similarly, while listening to others, people react differently.

This idea of three-dimensional observation is summed up in Figure 4.

Figure 4. Three dimension of observing a human being for determining prakriti.

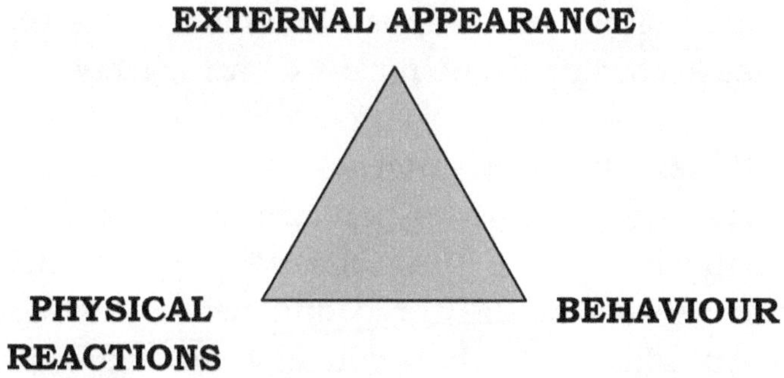

EXTERNAL APPEARANCE

PHYSICAL REACTIONS   **BEHAVIOUR**

Our internal and external being

All of us are aware of our external appearance and that is our identity for ourselves and for the world. To this particular appearance, a name is assigned or rather two or three names are given. That way, there is clarity about individuals and their identities. 'My' apparent individuality is asserted from my features like shape of my nose, lips, complexion, eyes and other features of the body. I am what I am in comparison to others. When we describe someone's appearance, we generally say things like big eyes, small eyes, sharp nose, small nose, flat nose or upturned nose, etc. Normally, we observe the external features of others quite spontaneously and naturally. In fact, we observe others more than ourselves as we see ourselves only for that brief time when we are standing in front of the mirror. It is interesting that many people do not know how they look from the side and some are quite surprised to see their side-pose from the photographs. Besides that, when we look at ourselves in mirror, it is always with indulgence and involvement. Thus, the perception of our outer appearance is visa vie others and also according to the norms of our society.

Prakriti is like the internal appearance of an individual and to learn to perceive that, you have to widen the horizon of your observation and include various aspects of the three dimensions mentioned above. In addition to that, you have to also broaden the sphere of your observation and extend it to other people around you. Expand your mind to look at people not only externally and superficially but also from the point of view of their prakriti. It is not the matter of knowing your prakriti once for all, but to learn to observe yourself constantly. Diversion from prakriti to vikriti (a state of being unwell but not sick) happens due to various internal and external factors and you have to get used to observing that in order to restore to prakriti. That is the reason that this observation should be like a habit with you and just like you observe yourself or others externally, you need to do the same in reference to prakriti and the related behaviour of various individuals. Secret of a healthy and long life with strength and vitality is to attend to the state of vikriti immediately and do the needful. For that, you have to train yourself to recognise, what I call 'the internal being' of an individual.

Learning to Observe

I will explain below some principal external features and suggest that you observe people around you in reference to these. Get into a habit of looking at the appearance and behaviour of an individual in a different manner than you are used to. Initially, do not do this observation with the idea of determining prakriti. Simply, make an effort to expand your observation.

1. Hair:
    a. rough and coarse or soft
    b. dense growth, thin growth or medium
Rough and course hair denote vata, dense growth is for kapha whereas thin growth signifies pitta.

2. Skin:
    a. dry
    b. smooth
    c. oily
Dry skin denotes vata, smooth kapha whereas oily skin is a sign for pitta.

3. Body temperature:
    a. hot
    b. cold and dry

c. cold and moist

Hot represents pitta whereas cold is either vata or kapha. Vata is dry and cold whereas kapha is moist and cold.

4. Body smell:
   a. strong and sometimes bad
   b. fleshy
   c. practically none

Strong body smell denotes pitta whereas fleshy smell is a sign of kapha. The vata dominant persons who have dry skin have practically no smell.

5. Nails:
   a. rough
   b. bright and pink
   c. whitish and smooth

Rough nails are a sign for vata dominance whereas bright and pink nails are of those who have more fire or pitta. Whitish and smooth nails are for kapha dominant persons.

6. Complexion:
   a. radiating
   b. rather dull
   c. clear and smooth

Pitta dominant individuals have a radiating or slightly pinkish complexion whereas a dull complexion denotes vata dominance. Kapha-dominant persons have clear and smooth complexion.

7. Eyes (colour of the retina):
   a. clear and white
   b. greyish and dull
   c. pink or reddish

White, dull and reddish represent the domination of kapha, vata and pitta respectively.

8. Body structure and face features:
   a. shape of the nose: sharp, fine or thick or in between
   b. shape of the body: delicate or well formed and stable

The ones with delicate features are pitta dominant whereas slightly thicker features denote the predominance of kapha. Vata dominating individuals fall somewhere in between.

9. Body movements:
   a. fast
   b. slow and stable
   c. varied

Kapha-dominant persons are slow and stable whereas vata dominant are fast. The dynamic but not excessively fast ones are pitta dominant individuals.

10. Way of talking:
   a. slow and with little gaps
   b. fast
   c. rapid and almost missing some words
   d. dynamic with good self-expression

Slow ones are kapha-dominant, fast ones are pitta-dominant and rapid ones are vata-dominant individuals. Dynamic with good self expression are generally a mixture of pitta and kapha.

11. Way of listening:
   a. with patience and attention and slow in grasping

    b. grasping very fast

    c. with impatience and sometimes completing your sentence, attention wandering

Kapha-dominating individual are good listeners whereas vata ones are impatient. Pitta-dominant individuals are quick to grasp.

12. Climbing up and down the stairs:

    a. very fast, almost leaving one step in between

    b. very slow and stable

    c. medium

    d. variable

Very fast ones are obviously vata dominating and those who are slow are kapha dominating. Medium or variable are with the predominance of pitta

13. Response to door bells and telephones:

    a. very rapid, almost with a jump and making oneself breathless

    b. stable but quite fast

    c. in a rather slow and sluggish manner

The ones who almost jump up with a telephone ring or door bell are predominant in vata and those who let the telephone ring several times before reacting are kapha-dominant. The ones who are stable but fast enough are with pitta-dominance.

14. Decision making:

    a. rapid and sometimes rash and impulsive

    b. very slow and sometimes changing one's mind

    c. variable but mostly thoughtful

Kapha-dominant individuals are always slow to decide. Rapid and rather too quick are the vata-dominating persons. Individuals with pitta predominance normally fall in between but are thoughtful in their decisions.

15. Emotional reactions:
    a. predominant in irritation and worry
    b. predominant in anger
    c. generally patient and gulp down emotions

Vata-dominating individuals tend to get irritated and they tend to worry whereas pitta ones have a tendency to get angry rather quickly. Kapha-dominating individuals have patience and tend to suppress their emotions.

Make it a habit to observe the above-mentioned features in persons in the family, at the workplace, amongst your friends or anybody you encounter in day-to-day life. Listen to people carefully when they talk about themselves and pay attention to the following features that will give you an insight into their physiological reactions or other allied features of their personality. From conversations and from the narratives of your colleagues, friends and acquaintances, you may be able to get some information at a slightly profounder level than in the above 15 points, which can be easily observed.

16. Stool:
    a. immediately after getting up
    b. after breakfast
    c. irregular and tendency to have constipation

Pitta-predominant individuals sometimes wake up in the morning because of an urge for stool. Kapha ones tend to have the urge after drinking something or after breakfast. Vata ones have rather irregular stool and have a tendency to get constipated.

17. Hunger and thirst:
    a. eats and drinks a lot
    b. sometimes a lot, sometimes little
    c. eats and drinks rather less and in stable quantity

Pitta-dominant individuals have a big appetite and they eat and drink a lot due to the dominance of fire element. Vata-dominating individual vary from one time to the other in their appetite whereas kapha persons eat and drink less.

18. Sleep:
    a. very profound and love to sleep
    b. needs less sleep and can keep awake easily
    c. variable and sometimes restless

Kapha-dominating individuals are sleep-loving whereas pitta-dominant persons can do with little sleep. The vata ones are variable and they may get restless sleep at times.

19. Reaction to weather:
    a. dislikes cold weather
    b. dislikes summer
    c. dislikes windy weather

Kapha-dominating individuals dislike cold weather, in particular cold and wet. Pitta-dominant individuals suffer easily when it is hot whereas vata ones are very sensitive to windy weather.

Amongst the above 19 points for observation, some are apparent and others are revealed by most people through their conversation. When you learn to observe people a little more than you are used to, you will begin to see another dimension of them. Train your mind for several months in this direction. This observation should be done without thinking of any results or conclusions from it. This is the first step for the formation of a habit to observe.

Interpreting and Inferring the Observations

Once you see that you have become better at observing people around you and yourself as well, try then to interpret all these observations together. You may begin with two or three persons who are closer to you and around you. But you should not ask them any questions. This is a part of your training that you should be able to gather enough observation from external appearances of people and what they reveal about themselves through their conversation.

Any individual observation, if not seen in conjunction with all other related observations and not interpreted in its proper context, may lead to the wrong conclusion. The following examples will help you to sort out your information about determining the prakriti of your chosen cases. Try and choose few cases for your training which are quite different from each other.

Before I begin with different case studies, let me remind you of the following three important points:

- Vata and kapha are cold.
- Pitta is hot.

- The difference between vata and kapha is that vata is dry cold and kapha is wet cold.

Case 1: A person is slow and stable in body movements, lets the telephone ring several times before picking it up and does the same with the door bell. She or he takes always plenty of time to decide. This person has clear and smooth skin, clear eyes and lots of hair. He or she eats and drinks in a limited quantity. Generally, this person loves to sleep and feels tired if the weather is wet and cold. This person has well-connected joints and ligaments. Persons of this category generally postpone things to be done to the next day and that is why their offices and homes are not very well organised.

*This is a clear case of a **kapha** prakriti.*

Case 2: Always complaining of heat, this person sweats a lot and tends to smell bad at times. He/she eats and drinks in plenty but is not fat. Skin is not smooth and gets pimples from time to time but the complexion is bright. Hair growth is not dense. Some of this category may tend to lose hair. This person has plenty of energy. He or she is rather impatient, especially before meals. Persons of this category have a tendency to get easily angry.

*This is a clear case of a **pitta** prakriti.*

Case 3: Speaking and walking rapidly, swift in their actions, these individuals are quick to decide. They are disturbed with windy weather and their complexion is rather dull. Skin gets dried up very quickly and they need to use a lot of oil in dry weather. They get easily irritated and are quick to show emotions like fear, anxiety, etc. They are intolerant to cold and shiver easily. They have usually prominent blood vessels.

*These are the **vata** prakriti persons.*

The Mixed Prakriti

After the three major types of individual constitutions, we turn to other types, which are constituted by the combination of two principal energies. When there is mixed prakriti, an individual may have some traits of both these. This will also be evident from the outward appearance. For example, a thick hair growth (kapha factor) but not a smooth skin as a kapha-dominant person will have. The eyes are not clear white but pinkish. When we come to the personality traits and physical reactions of the persons with mixed prakriti, they have traits of two types. Let us see some case studies for mixed prakriti.

Case 4: This person is quick to react and decide and is rather rapid in movements. With all these vata characteristic, this person also has radiant complexion and has typical reddish eyes a pitta dominant person would have. This person is very sensitive to food products which are hot in their Ayurvedic qualities like sour and spicy stuff and tends to get pimples or herpes. Some parts of the body are oily like the back and face but arms and legs are dry. Tolerance to heat and cold varies with this person and tends to be angry and impulsive at times.

*This is a person with **vata-pitta** constitution.*

Case 5: With the thick growth of hair and clear skin, well formed body structure, this individual may allude you to be a typical kapha-dominant type but you may feel that he/she is rather rapid in movements and quick to decide. Look very carefully in the eyes of this person with a smoky appearance and that is indicative of the vata aspect of prakriti. It may be a reverse situation where skin and hair may give an appearance of a vata-dominant person but the eyes are clearly indicating the dominance of kapha. This individual may give you an impression of being rather contradictory in her/his nature; at times quiet and tolerant whereas at other times, quite a contrast to that.

*This is an individual with **vata-kapha** constitution.*

Case 6: Here is an individual with fine features and a delicate built but with dense hair growth and clear skin and clear eyes. Contrary to these features, we have an individual with well-formed and strong body, less hair, radiant complexion and slightly reddish eyes. You will notice that the individuals of this category can be tolerant but at times or when provoked, they may explode like a volcano. This person may have phases of eating and drinking a lot, and in contrast to that, may consume very little food and drinks. Imagine that you have known someone who ate a lot when you invited her/him over and six months later, this individual may eat half the quantity when you had specifically made big portions for this person. These individuals are at times over-dressed in winter and at other times may be enjoying the cold weather.

*This is an individual with **pitta-kapha** prakriti.*

Case 7: Here is an individual who can adjust to most situations and generally gives an appearance of being well balanced and contented. He/she is able to maintain equilibrium in odd and difficult situations. The skin is smooth like that of a kapha person but has also the radiance of pitta. Rapidity of vata is balanced with the stability of kapha. This individual's body is capable of maintaining equilibrium in diverse weather conditions and other external circumstances. This individual has good stamina and immunity.

*This person has **samadosha prakriti** (equilibrium of all the three energies).*

Prakriti and Pulse in Ayurveda (Prakriti)

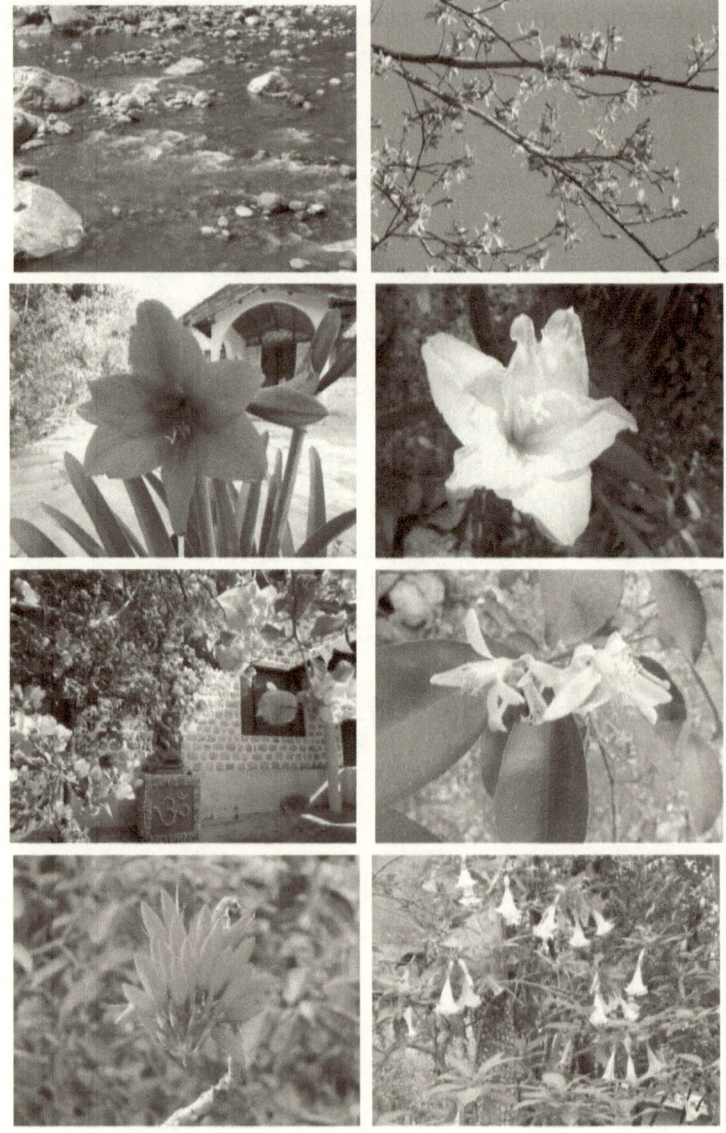

3

Infinite Variations in Prakriti

In the previous chapter, seven types of prakriti have been described. However, there are infinite variations of prakriti as diverse other factors have to be taken into consideration.

It is relatively easy to understand and to be able to determine the prakriti of people or of your own as far as you limit yourself to seven types. However, there are many other factors essential to the seven major types of prakriti, and you will realise that with these variations in each of the above types, we will arrive at a countless number of potential prakriti. But if you have learnt the first major step and have developed the ability to determine the seven major types as distinct from each other, the rest will be easier for you. We will now examine the factors that provide further diversity.

1. **Fundamental energy or *ojas*:** There are variations of the fundamental vitality, stamina and immunity from one person to another. Let us take an example of ten persons of samadosha prakriti. All of them may show differences despite being in harmony. They may be different in their fundamental energy levels. Think of that

55

in finer details and imagine them at a scale of from 0.1 to 10. Thus, you have one hundred factors in samadosha. We can apply the same to other six types and we already have numerous types of individuals. To understand this in a more concrete sense, think of the three energies in the form of blocks. In one of the samadosha prakriti person, one block of each energy is present. It could be possible that in another samadosha person, two blocks of each of the energies (vata, pitta and kapha) are present. Like this, let us imagine that there are individuals with up to 10 blocks of each energy. The person with 10 blocks of energy will have the highest of ojas (immunity and vitality). Thus, the fundamental energy quantitatively varies in different human beings.

2. **Degree of dominance:** In the above cases, there are several features to denote the dominance of a particular dosha. It is quite possible that an individual may not have all these characteristics but only some of them. It is also possible that some of these characteristics may be more prominent than the others. All these denote the degree of dominance of that particular vital energy. For example, you know a person who worries a lot. Start noticing the other features described for vata and you will realise that you will find several of these features quite evident in this person. On the other hand, there can be a person who 'tends to worry' and the other allied features may be there to a lesser degree. Thus, there are variations in the degree of dominance of a dosha from one individual to another.

3. **Different proportions in mixed prakriti:** There are three types of mixed prakriti but the proportion of each of the two dominant dosha may vary. For example, in a person with vata-pitta prakriti, the two energies may be present in any proportion. If there is more pitta than vata, we can call it a pitta-vata prakriti. Imagine the similar variations in vata-kapha and pitta-kapha types or prakriti. The proportion of the two doshas may also vary at different stages of one's life. For example, in a vata-pitta person, the pitta energy may be more pronounced at youth whereas the vata energy may take bigger proportion after the middle age.

Just like millions and billions of people on this earth can be distinguished from each other on the basis of their external features, the same is true for their inner being or prakriti. You should consider the prakriti of a person like his or her inner face. Keep in mind the seven major types of prakriti and allow for some variations in them. With practice, your horizon will gradually enhance and you will be able to spontaneously observe people for their prakriti as you now see and distinguish them outwardly.

Prakriti and three Gunas

It has been already stated that an individual has six dimensions of being at physical and mental levels and the seventh dimension is the soul or the energy that enliven these six dimensions. The three doshas (vata, pitta and kapha) and three gunas (rajas, sattva and tamas) mutually influence each other. To learn well about prakriti and vikriti and from reverting back from vikriti to prakriti, you need to understand the interaction of the guna and dosha. But first of all, let us discuss the influence of your state of mind on your prakriti.

Rajas guna is the activity of the mind and we use that during our daily routine for organising, planning, performing our functions for our livelihood and survival. Rajas is the state of mind full of activity that involves our five senses. The activity has a saturation point and senses and mind are fatigued. The hindered by the state of tamas where activity stops and there comes a state of immobility or inaction of the mind. The night time is the time of tamas. We sleep and the mind comes in a state of tamas. During sleep, senses are partially closed and mind does not acquire any new knowledge. It is important to know here that tamas also includes those activities of the mind which hinder mental development. Thoughts like jealousy, competition, anger, excessive attachment to material goods and people, etc. are some example that hinder the development and brings one in tamasic state of mind.

The third guna, sattva is the state of stillness of the mind. It is a spiritual state when we bring the mind to a total rest. Sattva is a state of purity when our mind is silenced and gets away from the activities of the world. At this state, the mind has oneness with the soul or the immense source of energy, which is our cause of being. Those of you have studied yoga may know that sattva leads to a yogic state of mind.

In day to day life, sattva helps balance our rajas and tamas. The balance in three qualities of the mind is important to maintain health. A hectic state of mind and over activity leads to an imbalance of vata, and too much tamas that involves lack of action, movement and too much sleep leads to an imbalance of kapha. Similarly, kapha imbalance leads to a tamasic state of mind and vata imbalance leads to hectic state of mind. Imbalance of pitta may lead to anger and thus a tamasic mental state. Direct relationship of pitta and kapha should be understood as is the energy at the physical level and energy at the subtle level respectively.

In the present context of prakriti, a balanced and sattvic person may delude you to judge her/his prakriti. For example, you may notice with affirmation all external signs of pitta prakriti in a person but may be confused with his/her patience, calm. My students in the past have tried to look for kapha prakriti as well in such a case but were confused not to find any sign of that. Thus, it is important also to pay attention to the sattvic qualities of a person while considering prakriti. Another example of that is a kapha or vata prakriti person may look radiating due to sattva or yogic power and that may be confusing for you for a pitta prakriti symptom. A person with too much tamas may give an appearance of total lack of energy and may confuse you in prakriti determination. Similarly, a person of kapha prakriti, when forced into hectic life may give you an impression of vata prakriti, which actually may be a vata vikriti due to a forced lifestyle contrary to the basic nature of this particular person.

Prakriti and Vikriti Confusion

This is one factor that confuses people and many therapist the most in prakriti determination. In nineties, there were branches of a big centre of Ayurveda in Western Europe and they brought young therapists from India to fascinate people with prakriti determination. However, these young and inexperienced persons mostly gave a wrong diagnosis to people. I realised that in my weekend seminars in Germany and Switzerland when almost everybody said that they had vata prakriti. Compared to India, the lifestyle in Europe was such that everybody appeared having vata prakriti to these young therapists.

Always remember that prakriti is a state of balance and despite the dominance of one or two dosha or energies, it is the state of health. It is you and your natural being. Health is to maintain one's prakriti and when it diverts from its natural path, take an immediate action to restore it.

We will discuss more of this theme in the vikriti section to make sure that you do not confuse the state of prakriti with vikriti.

Some Interesting Experiences with Prakriti

My experiences in Ayurveda seminars in Europe may be useful to state here as they might help you clarify some doubts that may arise after having read the above description.

Ayurveda has become very popular during the last decade particularly in German-speaking countries. There are some schools which have sprung up to provide some training for a month or two and then these 'graduates' teach or even practise. Evidently, these 'teachers' or 'practitioners' acquire very superficial knowledge of the subject. We in India say that one need several lives to learn the wisdom of Ayurveda. One of the beliefs of some such schools is to glorify certain types of prakriti and to condemn the other types. This wrong notion is further propagated when other people learn that from teachers trained with this notion.

A young lady who is teaching Ayurveda and yoga in Germany invited me to do a one-week seminar with her and her students. She herself was convinced that pitta is the best prakriti and that is why she is a brilliant and a charming person. Kapha prakriti was downgraded in her opinion and she thought these people were slow and are a drag and perhaps also not so intelligent. In this seminar, I told her that she had a pitta-kapha prakriti and that was almost unacceptable for her. It took me several days to completely convince her of the rational basis the kapha features predominant in her body and personality. This poor lady was quite unaware that the great Albert Einstein also had pitta-kapha prakriti.

Variations in the universe do not mean that certain things are good or bad. There are varied colours, smells, vegetations, seasons, and so on. We should look at the prakriti or the individual constitution in a similar manner. The great factor in a creative genius is not what prakriti he or she has. It is the fundamental energy that plays a great role. Each type of prakriti amongst the seven fundamental types has its own specific characteristics. The same basic quality can be used for a positive or negative purpose. For example, dominance of fire element can be used for creative purpose or it can find its outlet in the form of anger. Air and ether elements may be used to expand oneself in terms of experience and wisdom or to acquire a thoughtless rapidity that ultimately turns out to be negative. Stability of the water and earth elements can be used to solve the intricate problems or it can be just wasted by diminishing one's mobility or being lazy.

In a seminar elsewhere in Germany, the organiser was convinced that kapha prakriti was the best and that people with this prakriti were blessed with longevity. In another seminar, when I gave examples of different types of prakriti from amongst the students, one young lady started crying and said that I should not have revealed that before everybody. Many a times in such situations, people took prakriti as some kind of ailment or initial symptoms of an ailment. This attitude has now changed over the years with a constant spread of Ayurveda.

A friend of mine in Germany is ready to accept anything that is based on rationality and has some scientific basis. He was rather conservative in his view of the medicine and science that came from the orient but was extremely impressed when I told him about his prakriti and various physical and personality factors based upon that. What impressed him the most was the inter-link between various aspects of his character related to the element fire; to name a few—his reddish complexion, his anger, his brilliance and his resistance to cold.

In a weekend seminar, after I devote half a day on the theme of prakriti with practical demonstrations, there are always persons who come to me and tell me a story about their prakriti. Generally it is that they got themselves 'diagnosed' from someone or through questionnaires from a book but they were not convinced with that diagnosis.

It is better not to know your prakriti than to have a wrong idea about yourself. It is more reliable to try and do your own analysis with your own wisdom or seek the help of an appropriate Ayurvedic physician than to consult a person with little knowledge. It is not all that difficult to learn to analyse prakriti and in your own case it is the easiest. I have summarised below in Figure 5 the steps we have gone through to acquire the knowledge about prakriti.

Prakriti and Pulse in Ayurveda (Prakriti)

It is not difficult to know your prakriti if you follow the process described above. Begin always by affirming your own prakriti, as for yourself you have all the data and there is less possibility of confusion. Follow always these step as described in the figure below.

Figure 5. Steps for identifying your prakriti

LEARNING TO OBSERVE

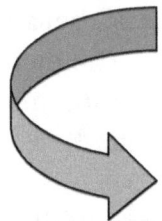

INTERPRETING THE OBSERVATION

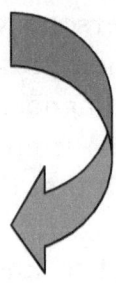

COMBINING THE OBSERVATION

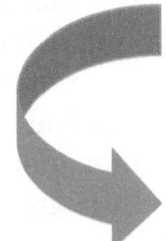

INFERRING THE OBSERVATION

4

Prakriti- a self organising system

It is important to learn that the bodily system has its perfect organisation and if this system is affected or attacked by external forces, it makes an effort on its own to reorganise and stabilise itself. The system makes every effort to revert back to its original nature. For example, if we get a small cut on the finger, it heals after some time. If we eat some bad food, body throws it out in one way or the other. If we feel cold, our body shivers to warm up itself. If it is hot, we sweat and the body cools down.

It is easy to understand this concept if you observe nature. The cosmos and the body are made of the same five fundamental elements. The body has an autonomous organisation which is similar to the cosmic organisation. When there are disturbances in nature due to too much rain, drought, storm, cyclones, excessive heat or cold, earthquake and so on, after a while, nature organises itself back to normality.

Deviation from prakriti

You have already learnt that deviation from prakriti is vikriti or a state of being unwell, which is not a sickness. You come to a state of feeling unwell and you cannot prescribe the reason for it. Sometimes it is not even the feeling of being unwell but a lack of one's optimum energy level. It is important to understand that you are liable to get a vikriti of your dominating dosha or doshas from factors such as weather, unbalanced nutrition, change of place, overwork, too much travelling or emotional factors, and so on. Actions which do not coordinate with the external environments vitiate other doshas also which are not dominant iy your prakriti. For example, even if your prakriti is not vata but the weather is extremely windy and you eat cold food and sleep very little or are travelling, it is probable that you would get vata vikriti. The same effect could take place due to geographical change and not living according to that change of environment. For example, if you move from Delhi to Frankfurt where the winters are very cold and wet with very few sunny days and you do not alter your food habits and way of living, you may get kapha vikriti. You have to learn to stay active despite the weather and not eat excessively fatty and sweet diet. Many Indian immigrants to Western Europe or other cold countries stay too much indoors due to the wet, cold and dark weather. One has to learn to cover oneself well and go out despite the weather. Similarly, people from cold countries with few sunny days, stay too much in the sun when they are in countries, where the sun shines almost every day. There is an amusing old Indian saying to this effect: 'Only dogs and Englishmen go out on a summer afternoon'.

Everything in this universe is fluid and not rigid and so are our physical and mental reactions to the environment. The change from prakriti to vikriti will keep happening due to diverse factors. The role of Ayurvedic practice is to diagnose oneself with simple observations of the urine, stool, taste in the mouth, pulse, etc. and then take immediate action to help the body re-establish its prakriti.

The body itself is capable of reverting back from vikriti to prakriti. For example, if we eat too many pitta-promoting things and get too much heat in the body, mild diarrhoea may occur to get rid of excessive heat from the body. If we consume something that is hard to digest or is spoilt, our body throws it out to regain its balance. In such cases, you should not take any medication to hinder the process of nature and let the events take their own course. Body has a perfect system and our intervention should be to helping nature. In case of a diversion from prakriti, we should help the process of recovery by taking appropriate measures like balanced food, rest, massage, baths and other such simple measures. Due to an external attack of bacteria or viruses or due to an injury, prakriti deviates to vikriti. In such cases, first of all appropriate medication and a proper diet are required for healing and then the body gradually reverts back to its natural state.

Prakriti and vikriti

Your prakriti is your body's basic nature and the tendency of the nature is to be orderly and healthy. Due to external factors like weather, climate, stress, wrong nutrition, etc., prakriti may change into vikriti or imbalance, which is a state of being unwell but not really a sickness. Vikriti is marked by the presence of subjective symptoms of being unwell.

Nature of the body is such that it reverts back to its natural conditions on its own. But if the factors disturbing this nature are very strong and constantly oppress it, the state of vikriti prolongs. We need appropriate food, drugs and other measures to revert back to prakriti. However, if the state of imbalance is left unattended for a long time, it will give rise to ailments or disorders.

It is normal to change from the state of prakriti to vikriti due to so many reasons in our day-to-day life. A normal healthy person automatically reverts back to prakriti. However, if you assist nature in her task, the process to revert back to prakriti will be rapid. Charaka, the great Ayurvedic sage from 6th Century B.C. had compared it to a fallen person after hitting a stone. The person will get up anyway; however, if someone gives him/her a hand, it is helpful.

Prakriti 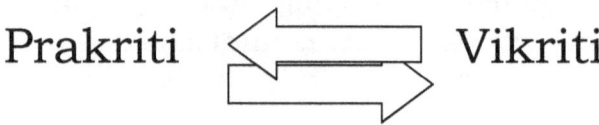 Vikriti

You can recognise the vikriti by various symptoms. These are mostly 'subjective symptoms'. Always remember that you are the best judge of your body. No machine and no physician can know your body better than you yourself. Thus do not ignore yourself and be always alert to the slight changes taking place in your body and state of mind.

Following table sums up the lists of symptoms you get due to vikriti in your three energies, which can upset your whole system. You may have one or more symptoms of vitiation. It is not essential that you have all the symptoms simultaneously. More intensive the vikriti, more are the symptoms. But your aim should be to nip the evil in the bud, react immediately at the slightest derangement from prakriti.

VATA	PITTA	KAPHA
*You get up in the morning with a stiff body.	*You perspire too much and have a body odour.	*You do not want to get up in the morning.
*You have often constipation or hard and dark coloured stool. Urine is grey or muddy.	*You get yellow to dark yellow urine and thin stool.	*You have a heavy feeling and wish to sleep the whole day.
*Your skin is too dry despite the fact you often oil it.	*You get reddish eyes.	*You feel drowsy during the day.
	*Your complexion looks reddish	*You get whiteness in urine, eyes and faeces.
*You have dull and ashy comp-	and with either skin eruptions	*You get whitish complexion

lexion and smoky eyes. *You get very often a dried throat and feel like drinking even during the night. *You have restless sleep or have trouble sleeping. *You yawn often and also suffer from hiccups. *You have fatigue that goes away after rest and sleep or hot bath. *You have intolerance and lack of endurance. *You feel often irritated and impatient.	or pimples. *You have abnormal hunger and thirst. Excessive eating does not make you fat. *You have often minor stomach related problems. *You get often pimples, herpes or blisters or tearing of the skin. *You feel excessive heat in your body. *You feel dissatisfied. *You get often bouts of anger.	without any glow and skin remains moist. *You have a sweet taste in mouth. You get excessive salivation. *You get often a cold sensation. *You get itchy feeling in your throat. *You get nausea from time to time. *You have a sense of lassitude. *You get inertness and depression at times.

From the above description, you will be able to find out when prakriti diverts and changes to vikriti. There are certain things in the description of vikriti that you may be already experiencing but may not necessarily think that they signify a diversion from your state of health. Some examples are hiccupping, yawning, sweet taste in mouth, undue anger and irritation, pimples or change in your complexion.

Once you understand scientifically the entire system of Ayurveda, you will realise the interconnection between the nagging problems you have and the balance of three main energies of the body. Imagine one morning, your stool is hard and dark. During the day you feel fatigued and yawn. If you catch these minor symptoms there and then, and do something, you will be fine by next day. However, if you ignore, next morning you will have slightly stiff body upon getting up and despite the night's rest, you will feel tired. This state will also affect your external appearance and you may find that you have a dull appearance. You will see that if you will take measures to treat vata vikriti, all the symptoms that make you feel unwell will disappear. However, if you do not take measures and let this state go on, it will spoil the internal environment of your body and you will get a dull appearance over a period of time. In the long run, you may get sleep disturbances, various aches and pains, blood related ailments, and so on. It is important that you become conscious about your state of health and its relationship with your appearance and immediately find out the state of vikriti. Finding that you have diverted from state of health to non-health, you need to take measures to restore health without delay.

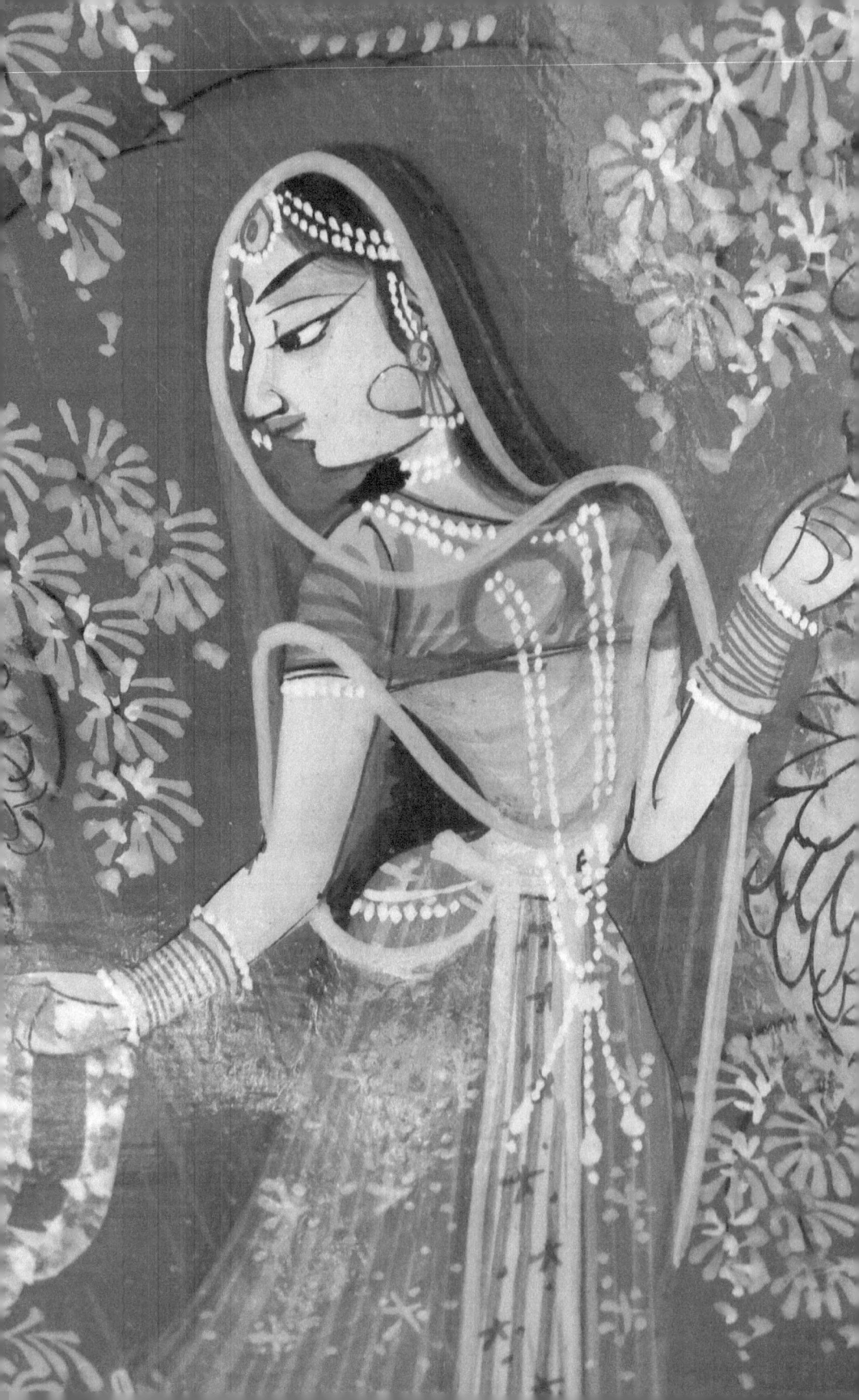

5

Relationship of Prakriti to Health and Disease

We have already talked about the self organisation of prakriti and its reversal in a natural way from vikriti to prakriti. However, if we human beings can help in this task of maintaining prakriti, we remain healthy and disease free. On the contrary, if we do anti-natural things and enhance and prolong the state of vikriti, we are get ill health and a short life span. If vikriti becomes chronic, it leads to ailments.

The biological aspect of vikriti

Vata, pitta and kapha are the three energies that are responsible for all the mental and physical functions of the body. They work in coordination with each other. For example, the function of vata is distribution of energy in the body. The formation of energy is the function of pitta by digesting food. For the digestion of food, we need digestive juices. Digestive juices are produced by kapha. They are carried from one place to another by vata. Once the energy is produced by pitta, vata distributes to each and every part of the body. If the quality of the digestive juices is not good or pitta is sluggish to perform its functions or vata is too quick or too slow, the total system is disturbed. You can compare this to the postal system. You are waiting for a letter from a friend. You ask your postman everyday if there is a letter for you. He has none. A letter sent by post is a collaborative work of so many people at different destinations and postman can give you only what he was given to deliver. For a letter to reach its destination, everybody related to this task should perform his/her function properly. Similarly, if someone has cold hands and cold feet, the error can be at the level of the quantity of energy (pitta), faulty distribution (vata) or digestive juices low in their quantity and quality (kapha).

Vikriti or the diversion from normal and natural is under or over function of one of the three energies, lack of coordination in the functions of the three energies or their displacement. The examples of under and over-functions of vata are low and high blood pressure. Under function of pitta is indigestion and heartburns or acidity denote displacement or over function. Excessive sleep and drowsiness is over function or displacement of kapha. Lack of secretions is an under-function of kapha.

Your dry skin is due to under function of kapha and over function of vata. Excessively oily skin is over function of pitta. Excessively moist skin is an over function of kapha. Under function of pitta will make you look pale whereas over function will give you reddish skin, pimples, skin irruptions, etc. Excessive vata makes your skin rough and dry.

Restoring Vikriti to Prakriti

Restoring vikriti to prakriti is the first duty of an individual towards his or her being. It is called svadharma. According to Ayurveda, the first priority of life should be health as when health is gone, all other is meaningless. In other words, it is also said that the body is the temple of soul. Soul is the infinite energy and cause of being. How can we keep the temple disorderly and dirty?

If vikriti remains unattended for a long period of time, it becomes chronic and takes the form of an ailment or disorder. I describe below in brief the measures to revert back to prakriti from vikriti. This is cited from my book, *Programming your Life with Ayurveda*. For more details, please consult my books, *Ayurveda: A way of Life, Ayurveda for Inner Harmony* and *Programming your Life with Ayurveda*.

Treatment of vata vikriti

- Drinking hot water is a remedial measure for vata vitiation. It is even better if you can boil one litre of water with three-four cardamoms and keep that water in a thermos to drink hot whenever you are thirsty.

- Do the oil saturation massage with warm oil. Go on applying warm oil on all parts of your body until the body does not take any more. For more details, please consult my book *Programming your Life with Ayurveda*.

75

- Take warm bath, dry fomentation and appropriate rest.

- Eat warm and unctuous food predominant in sweet and sour rasas. Avoid pungent, astringent and bitter substances. (For more details on nutrition, please consult my book *Ayurveda Food Culture and Recipes*).

- Take only hot foods and drinks and avoid all cold foods and drinks except fruits and salads.

- Recommended foods are milk, banana, papaya, citrus fruits, carrots, turnips, fenugreek (methi), kalonji, cumin, fennel, dill, cardamom and ginger.

- To cure vata vikriti, take herbal tea with basil pepper and liquorice. Add 4-5 basil leaves, half-teaspoon of powdered liquorice and a pinch of pepper (3 grains) in half litre water. Bring it to boil and let it cook for about five minutes on a low fire with the lid on. Put off the fire and let it stay like this for a few minutes. Filter and drink it.

- If your vata vikriti is caused due to an exposure to cold and you have stiffness and body ache, boil 6-7 crushed cardamoms and 7-8 leaves of basil in half litre water for five minutes. Keep the preparation covered and cook on a low fire. Drink it in two doses. You may add some candy sugar in it for taste.

- If you are suffering from fatigue due to vata, take

an herbal tea with big cardamom, clove and cinnamon. Crush one big cardamom, three cloves and a small piece of cinnamon and boil these in half litre water. Let it cook covered on low fire for about five minutes. You may add some candy sugar into it to sweeten. This preparation can also be taken as normal tea or chai with the addition of black tea and milk into it.

- Ajwain or thyme tea is also good to alleviate vata vitiation. Dose for ajwain or Thyme is half a teaspoon in half a litre of water. Make the tea as described above.

- Ginger, basil and cardamom tea is very effective in vitiated vata. Crush about 3 cubic centimetres of ginger, 5 basil leaves and 3 cardamoms. Add all this in half a litre of water and make the tea in a similar manner as has been described above. In case you do not have fresh ginger, replace it with half teaspoon of powdered ginger. Add some candy sugar in the end to make the spicy taste of the ginger milder.

- For treating vata imbalance, take one clove of garlic daily, crush it and add ¼ of a teaspoon of ghee and swallow it. Do not drink anything cold after taking this preparation.

- Crush one teaspoon each of kalonji and cumin along with two teaspoons of candy sugar. Split this into six doses and take three times a day for two days. If you think that you are still not completely cured from the symptoms of vata vitiation, repeat this for another few days.

- If your vata vitiation is too frequent and intense, you should take the treatment for 15 days or more with chaturbeej churan (powder of four seeds). Powder the following four different kinds of seeds in equal quantity: fenugreek, ajwain, cress and kalonji. Take half a teaspoon of this powder 3 to 4 times a day.

Treatment of pitta vikriti

Take the following measures to bring the vitiated pitta to equilibrium:

- Drink plenty of water, cold milk and cooling sherbets like brahmi or sandalwood.

- Take a cold bath and apply cooling ointments like sandalwood paste, ghee or coconut oil on your body. If you have burning sensation in a specific part of the body, you may apply sandalwood paste only on that specific part of the body.

- Take mud treatment. Yellow and fine variety of earth is used for this purpose. It is also called 'healing earth' or 'Multani mitti' in India. Make a thin paste with this earth by adding water and do an anointing with it on all over your body (*lepa*). Leave it for about half an hour and wash it off. This treatment will also make your skin smooth.

- Take foods that are dominant in sweet, bitter and astringent rasas. Suggested foods are rice, masoor dal, spinach, carrots, cabbage, pumpkin, courgette, aubergine, bitter gourd, dates, bananas, sweet apples and grapes, papaya, cold milk, ghee, fresh cheese (paneer), fennel, clove, coriander and liquorice.

- Take herbal teas like wormwood, neem, coriander and liquorice. Take extremely bitter substances only in a very moderate quantity. Use a few leaves of neem or wormwood and mix them with some ajwain to make the tea. The reason for this is that exclusively bitter rasa may cure your vitiated pitta but in turn may vitiate your vata. Equilibrium of drugs is important in Ayurvedic pharmacology.

- Take a teaspoon of juice of bitter gourd (*karela*) two times a day to pacify the excessive heat in the body.

Treatment of Kapha Vikriti

To reverse the state of kapha vikriti into your natural state or prakriti, take the following measures:

- Use spices like ginger, garlic, dill seeds, kalonji, fenugreek and mustard seeds.

- Take always freshly prepared hot food.

- Hot bath and vapour bath are very effective in

curing kapha vikriti. Force yourself to do physical exercise and go for walks.

- Make an effort to keep awake (less sleep).

- Make an effort to go out, meet people rather than sitting alone and feeling drowsy.

- Avoid watching too much television.

- Suggested foods are Soya beans, potatoes, cress salad, tomatoes, cauliflower, peaches, plums, citrus fruits and honey. Ghee should be avoided and cooking should be done in moderate quantity of sesame or olive oil. Sugar and products containing sugar should not be taken. To sweeten tea or coffee, use candy sugar.

- Take a clove of garlic everyday with some honey.

- Take herbal tea with ginger, cardamom, pepper and basil.

Conclusion

Prakriti determination is the precious wisdom from the ancient Vedic sages. It not only denotes the fundamental human constitution but it is also the basis of Vedic psychology. The prevalent mechanistic world view which is also applied in modern medicine treats all human beings at power and there is no concept of basic human identity. Same things are expected from everybody and the modern psychology is also based upon these fundamentals. However, the wisdom of prakriti teaches us to take into consideration the human variations and recognise the individual identity of each person. There should not be same expectations from the siblings or from all members of a particular group. The application of the wisdom of prakriti can pave way for a better understanding at familial and social levels and help make congenial atmosphere at work place for enhancing work efficiency. A better understanding of each other at different levels of the society can lead to peace and harmony.

Prakriti determination can help us to understand the aptitude of young children and help them find an appropriate work. Treating all children with the same measures and having same expectations from them in a family, at school or in other social situations proves to be cruel for them. Thus, wisdom of prakriti provides us space.

Prakriti and Pulse in Ayurveda (Prakriti)

In today's world the biggest contribution of prakriti is to use it as preventive method for warding off ailments. Diversion from prakriti to vikriti is like an alarming system in our body. Humanity can be trained to distinguish between an ailment and a state of vikriti. With mechanistic view of modern medicine, people live disconnected from their bodies. They run to doctors for a slightest of diversion from their routine life they are used to. The whole medical industry is profit oriented and is based upon causing fear in people. Knowledge of Ayurveda, in particular of prakriti, can make human beings aware that the body is a dynamic system and is a part of the vibrant and forceful cosmos. Like in the cosmos, there are also constant changes in our physical system and it is our basic duty (svadharma) to learn to deal with these changes to take care and keep ourselves healthy, energetic and in a joyful mental state. Our body is not a machine that we take it to a mechanic in case of breakdown. What we have to learn with the wisdom of prakriti is to do all so that we never come to a point of breakdown.

Wisdom of prakriti is precious to develop physical and mental strength and lead a life which is more aware and which can lead us to health, fearlessness and a state of contentment. Modern medical industry works by causing fear and subjecting humanity to all kinds of un-needed medical examinations with expensive machines and sell extremely expensive treatments. When we human beings learn to take our responsibility, be self-confident for maintaining our health and live fearlessly, we will need the modern medicine only for emergencies and not to treat cough, cold, allergy, fatigue and numerous other minor ailments. All this can change the economics of the health care system and can make people healthier and happier human beings.

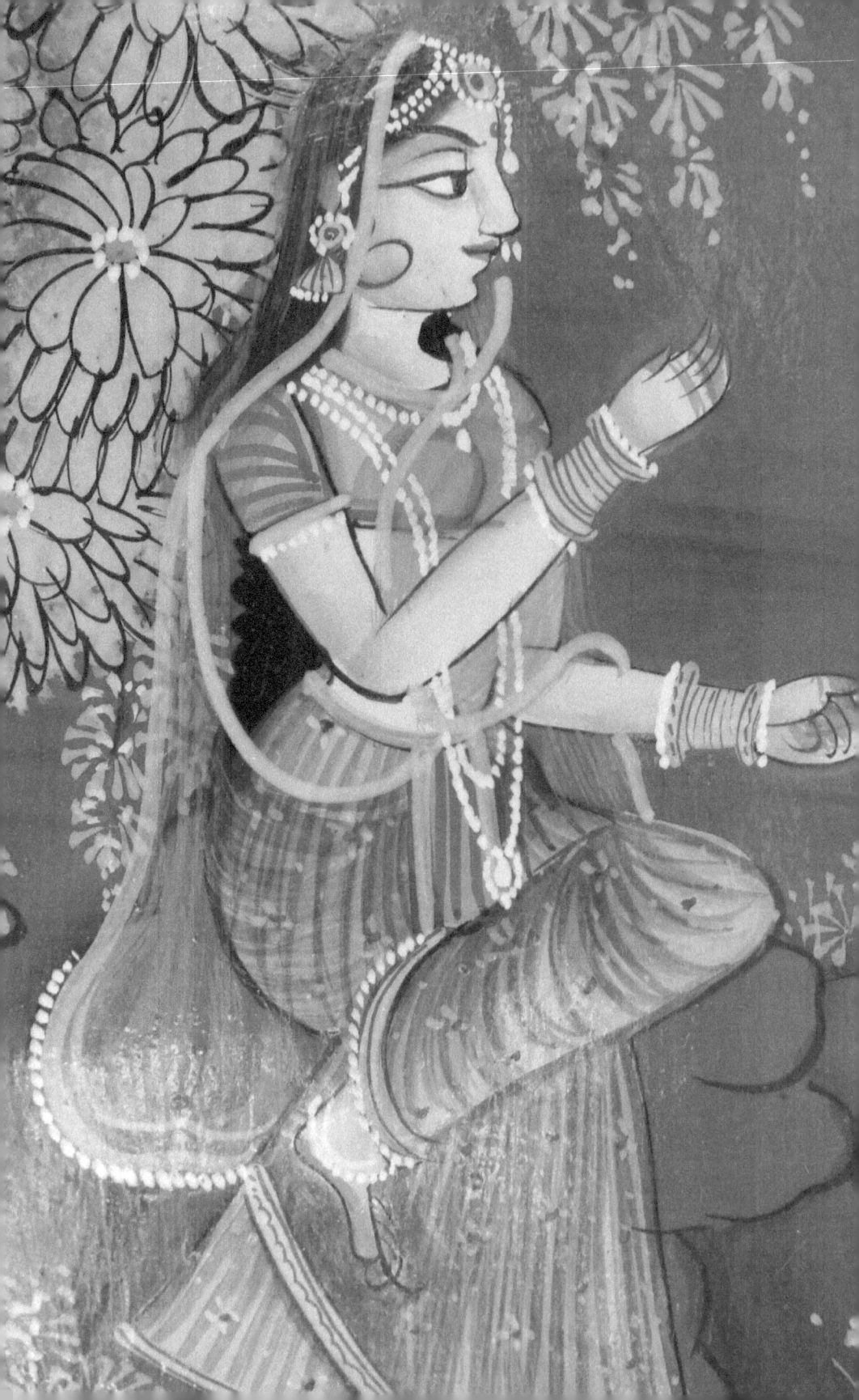

Part II
Nadi Priksha: The Pulse Diagnose

Prakriti and Pulse in Ayurveda (Pulse)

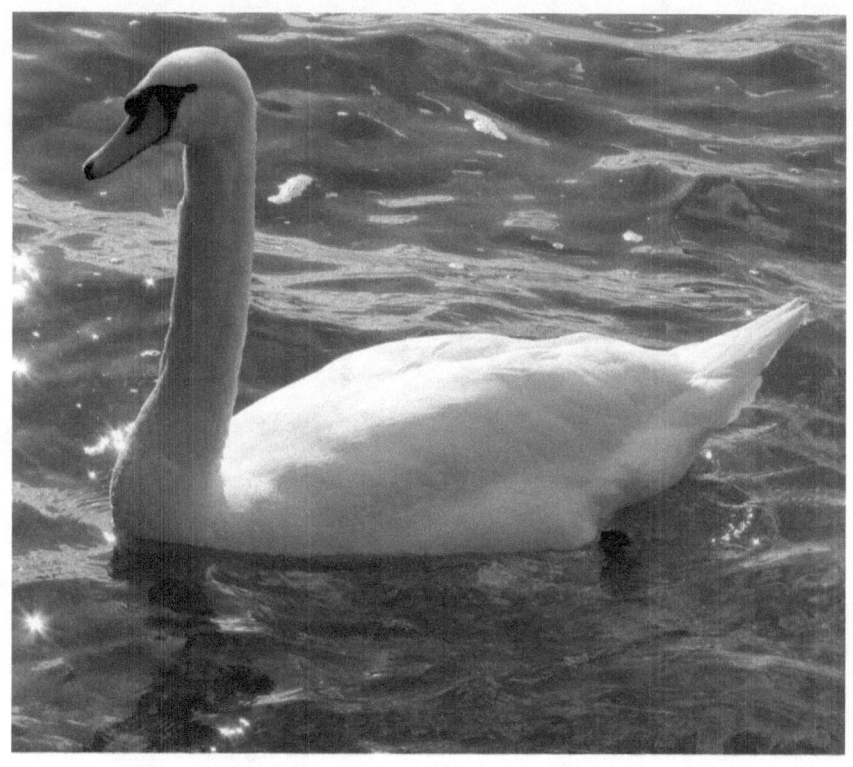

1

Pulse Diagnosis and Ayurveda

In the Vedic tradition, all disciplines of knowledge are systematized and that is also true for Ayurveda. Like in the other disciplines, in Ayurveda also, any new knowledge was assimilated after experimentation and after long time research to fit in with rest of the system. The ancient scholars were also very particular about the terminology of the new discipline. Interesting part of the Ayurvedic wisdom is that it always assimilated wisdom from all over the world and sometimes this knowledge was lost in their home countries but conserved in Ayurveda. This is particularly true about medicinal plants. At present, the plants in Ayurveda are imported from all over the world.

Pulse diagnosis is not a part of the scriptural tradition of Ayurveda but was integrated into it later, probably around 3 Century AD. However, it seems that it was assimilated completely and officially into the system around 5-6 Century AD. A sacred quality of the Vedic tradition is that once a discipline is accepted into a particular system, it is protected and conserved. In fact, this is the only tradition in the world which has been conserved unaltered in many aspects since antiquity.

The integration of knowledge from outer sources into the Vedic tradition was always done over a long period of time but in such a perfect way that ultimately it did not seem foreign at all. The concepts or techniques were officially integrated into written scriptures only after they had been penetrated in the tradition for several hundred years and were already moulded in the tradition and customs of the country. Sages devised the appropriate terminology for new knowledge and wrote on its relationship to the fundamental Vedic thinking and thus, composing appropriate literature. The perfect tailoring of the concepts was to such an extent that a century later, it was hard to tell between the indigenous and foreign knowledge.

Pulse diagnosis, which is an integral part of Ayurvedic practice, has somewhat similar story. It is not a part of the Vedic tradition and nor was it mentioned by Charaka or Sushruta. It first appeared in the Ayurvedic literature from around 5-6 Century AD. Nevertheless, there are many Ayurvedic Acharyas who try to establish that the pulse examination is from Vedic times. I have discussed this theme in the next chapter to illustrate the origin of pulse diagnosis from the Chinese tradition. The descriptions of Ayurvedic pulse examination is very different as compared to the Chinese, but the origin of this idea that the pulsation of blood vessels carried unique information on our body system is most likely Chinese.

Exchange of knowledge between different cultures of the globe has always existed in human history. The only difference is that the pace was very much slower in the former times. I do not know whether Hippocrates ever met with Sushruta or his students, but following story shows that the scientific and medical wisdom of the world was integrated and synthesized from the times immemorial. I gave my basic book on Ayurveda to my French Professor, René Couteaux in 1992. Professor Couteaux was a European sage with a tremendous wisdom from the ancient civilisations. After reading the book, he told me about the striking similarity between the Ayurvedic wisdom described in my book and Aphorisms of Hippocrates he studied in nineteen hundred forties as a student of medicine in Paris. Later I learnt from the History of Medicine that Hippocrates, who lived on the island of Cos in Greek travelled a lot in Asia and had exchanged wisdom with Auyrvedic sages. Like Sushurata, Hippocrates also said that besides three principle energies, blood is almost like the fourth energy or dosha.

In our times when the world has become a cosmic village, it is time that we integrate the medical wisdom in such a way that the humanity can benefit maximum from the existing world wisdom.

I have written this part with an intension that the interested reader is able to learn not only the historical and other theoretical aspects of pulse examination but is also inspired to learn to practice this diagnostic method. For this reason, I have used the modern terminology for the explanations of the pulse variations in various conditions of health and disease. The classical terminology is mostly on the movements of animals. My argument is that if people do not have a direct experience of nature and have really not 'felt' those movements from animals over a long period of time, they would be unable to

Prakriti and Pulse in Ayurveda (Pulse)

comprehend the phenomenon of pulse. My experience in my Ayurvedic classes shows that students feel very good to use the similes of the animals but they are unable to technically apply them to learn pulse diagnosis. Thus, I hope the new terminology based on sound and rhythm would provide a better comprehension. In addition to that a nine-step programme for learning to examine the pulse for diagnosis will provide the reader an initiation into this wisdom. When the students are learning with me or another teacher, the key factor is the gradual practice over a long period of time to attain this knowledge. Learning to examine the pulse can be compared to learning concentration practices for the purpose of meditation. The master or guru can show you the way, but you must walk on your own.

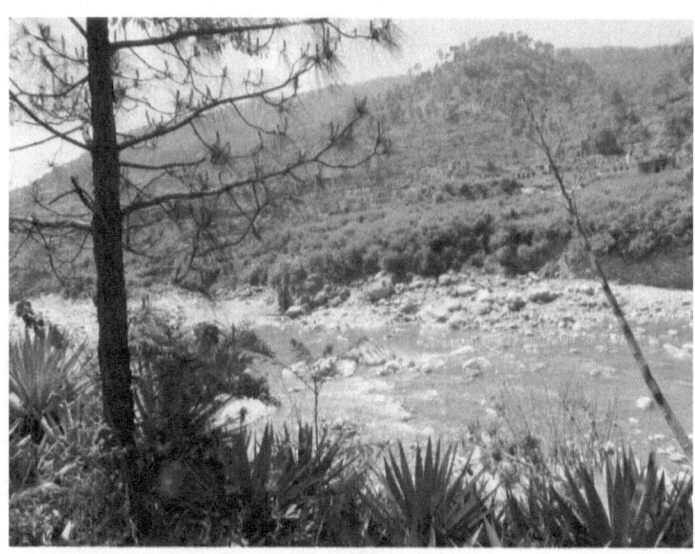

2
History of Pulse Diagnosis

Historical facts

The first written documents on pulse diagnosis are found during 5 Century AD. It means that pulse diagnosis existed many centuries before this, it was completely accepted by the Ayurvedic sages and integrated into Shastriya (scriptural) tradition. After its integration in the scriptural tradition of Ayurveda with its specific vocabulary, pulse diagnosis was unanimously accepted and became an integral part of the Ayurvedic tradition.

There are some Vaidyas (Ayurvedic physicians) and Acharyas (Auyrvedic sages) who are of the opinion that pulse diagnosis is from the Vedic period. However, historically this does not seem to be the fact. . Blood circulation, different energy points in the body and the extensive network of energy channels (that include also blood vessels) are described in the oldest written document on medicine— the Atharva Veda. There is a classification and different names are given to the major blood vessels in Atharva Veda. They are called Shira, Hira and Lohita.

During the period of Upanishads, the blood vessels are described in more details. The word 'nadi' is used

91

for the blood vessels in Prashno Upanishad where it is said that the heart has a hundred nadis, each one of them has hundred branches going to the body. Each one of the branch has further seventy two thousand branches. Thus, the whole body has seventy-two billion nadis through which the living element (blood) circulates in each and every part of the body.[*]

Similarly, there are descriptions of blood vessels in other scriptures as well. In *Charaka Samhita* and *Sushruta Samhita*, there are anatomical details of the body. Sushruta has described the anatomy in more details, as he was a surgeon. Dhamnis take the blood to the heart with force whereas Siras bring the blood back to the heart with lesser force. Sushruta has also described the special fragile areas in different parts of the body called Marmas[**]. A surgeon has to pay attention during surgery not to touch or hurt the marmas. Marmas are the points where blood vessels, nerves and ligaments cross together. If the marma points are attacked one way or the other, they disturb the functions of the sense organs such as speech, tactile sensation, taste, sight, etc. The mental state also gets deranged. The total number of marmas in the body is 107.

Despite all these anatomical details in the Vedic literature, where much importance is given to blood circulation through which prana or the living element of the body circulates everywhere, there is no mention of the methods of diagnosis through pulse

---

[*] *Prashno Upanishad*, Prashana 3.
[**] *Sushruta Samhita, sharirasthanam*, VI, 15.

examination. Nevertheless, the pulsation of the blood vessels was a known phenomenon. The pulsation is called spandan in scriptural tradition and it is written that it is an indicator of life. However, there is no description of the examination of pulsation for diagnosis or even the variations and diversity of spandan or pulsation. Thus, it sounds very reasonable to say that pulse examination did not exist in ancient India. It would be mere chauvinism to believe that the diagnostic method of pulse examination exists in India from the Vedic times.

Ayurvedic wisdom is not exclusively the historical documentation of ancient scriptures. Ayurveda has dynamically evolved through ages and new knowledge has been constantly incorporated into it. India had an active exchange of culture and medicine with the West since antiquity. There was an exchange of knowledge between the Ayurvedic sages and the great sage of medicine from the island of Cos in Greece, Hippocrates (460-377 BC). In the *Aphorisms of Hippocrates* there is something similar to prakriti or the individual constitution and the doshas. Two centuries later, Alexander the great with his entourage of physicians brought us tremendous wisdom of Greek medicine that was integrated into Ayurveda. Greek system of medicine was also adopted by Iraq and Persia and was integrated with their own systems of medicine. Ayurveda has integrated tremendous wisdom from the world through ages as well as Ayurvedic wisdom was inseminated throughout the world since ancient times. The fact that Ayurvedic products come from all over the world shows that we have taken medicinal wisdom from the whole world.

After the science of pulse examination was integrated into Ayurveda, there were two exclusive treatises on pulse examination:
1. *Nadi Pariksha* (Pulse Examination) by Ravana
2. *Nadi Vigyan* (Science of Pulse) by Kannada.

Besides these two treatises, the pulse examination is also included in different bodies of yoga and Ayurveda. *Sharngadhara Samhita, Bhava Prakasha* and *Yoga Ratnakar* are some major sources for the first written and scientifically oriented documents on pulse examination and its application in diagnostics.

It is likely that the pulse examination acquired popularity several hundred years before the literature was written on this theme. Perhaps it was integrated into the classical Ayurveda at a later date due to its immense spread and recognition. Since the pulse examination existed in China around 1000 century BC, it is reasonable to think that the it originated there. It seems likely that this wisdom first travelled to the West through Mongolia, where it was integrated into Arabic and Greek medical systems and then from there it came to us via Persia and Iraq. However, it was not the only route from where we got this wisdom. In the northwest India, we got this wisdom through Tibet as well. A very likely source seems to be through Buddhist Monks around the 9th century from Tibet. Buddhism was introduced into Tibet via China. After the adoption of Buddhism, there was more cultural exchange between Tibet and India and thus, also the doors opened for the exchange of scientific wisdom and Tibet became the gateway between the two big cultures of Asia.

The science of pulse examination was further developed on the Indian continent under the tantric and the Siddha tradition. Let us now see its rational basis in the context of Vedic thinking of which Ayurveda is a part.

Pulse diagnosis in reference to the Vedic cosmogony

The word 'nadi' originates from the word *nad*, which means a loud holy sound that is beyond any causative factor and is associated with the cause of being. In cosmogony, the first element of the five elements the cosmos is made of is 'nad'. It is also called *Nad Brahma*– the sound of creation. The vehicle of sound is the element akasha or space, which is the first causative factor of the phenomenal world as without space nothing can exist.

In yogic literature, there is a description of nad that exists in our body. By closing all senses, breathing and by concentrating on one's inner being, one hears the internal sound or nad. One experiences the body in totality with this sound. In my opinion, this sound is related to the blood flow and totality of the space of the body. Each one of you can experiment with this and get your own experience. However, before doing this practice, you need to have some experience in *pranayama* (control of the vital energy). This is

95

because you have to hold your breath for a little while and if you are not trained in pranayama, you may feel giddy or extremely out of breath after the practice.

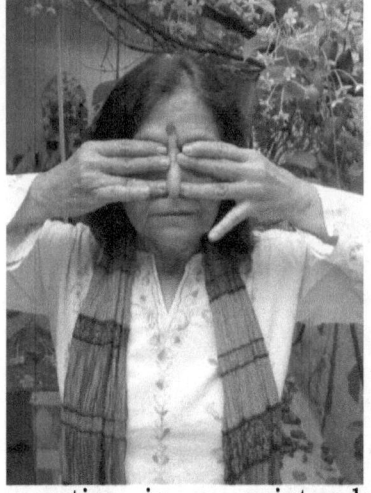

Close your ears with your thumbs, eyes with index and middle fingers and both nostrils with ring fingers as shown in the figure. Do for a short while in the beginning. Do the practice repeatedly so that you get used to applying appropriate pressure and holding the breath at the same time. Do this practice in a quiet place and during the silent moment of the day. Gradually you will begin to hear the inner sound of the blood flow and your heart beat. You will get a relationship with your inner spandan of the energy, which is the sign of being alive.

Nadi literally means a tubular structure but in anatomical sense, it is the tubular structure through which vital energy flows to all parts of the body. Nadi has *spandan* or pulsation. Although in ancient literature, there is no description of the *nadi pariksha* or the pulse diagnosis, nevertheless the pulsation or spandan is repeatedly called *pranadahini*– the life-giving. Thus, the importance of pulse and pulsation is in the sense of element space. Nadis have an extensive network and they reach each and every part of the body in a finest way. This is the reason that Ayurvedic sages integrated pulse examination into the traditional medical system of India.

Terminology used for pulse examination

In the historical accounts of pulse examination, it is important to understand some of the major terms which were used for explaining pulse examination. The pulse denoting the dominance of diverse doshas was compared to the movements of the animals. Similes of *sarpa* (snake), *hansa* (swan), *mayur* (peacock), *kaka* (crow), *manduka* (frog), etc. are frequently used.

There is also other terminology to describe the characteristics of the pulse. We can classify pulsation in five main categories and in each category, there are several words to describe the subtlety of pulsation. Following are the five major types with some example of other descriptive words for each category.

- Fast
- Medium slow
- Slow
- Heavy
- Specific

Fast: some terminology of this category is; *chapala, vegavati, vegavahini, teevra, atichapala, chapala-deergha, chala,* etc.
Medium slow: *sthira, stabdha, sthira-balavati, susthira, prithula, jada,* etc.

97

Slow: *mandaga, manda, ksheenagati, anusapanda, nishchala, mantharagati, shithila,* etc.
Heavy: *deergha, sukshma, krisha, prabala,* etc.
Specific: *trutita, atisheeta, ushana, gurvi, laghvivegavati,* etc.

I feel that the use of this ancient terminology will make the description in the present book very difficult to comprehend and therefore I am not giving the explanation of each of these terms. Language is always used in its cultural context. It is more practical to use the modern terminology for the present edition as this book is meant for the general reader all over the world.

Pulse examination in modern India

Pulse examination is an important and almost essential part of the Ayurvedic diagnosis in today's India. In fact, a patient will not be happy if he or she went to a vaidya and the pulse was not examined. Seeing the popularity of pulse examination in Europe where Ayurveda has become popular only since two decades, I feel that pulse examination speaks for a special connection between the doctor and the patient. The doctor examines the pulsation of the blood and the blood travels in each and every part of the patient's body. I often say jokingly that pulse examination 'establishes a blood relationship between the doctor and the patient'. It is very amusing that when people call me for an appointment for a private session in Europe, they question me straight away if I will examine their pulse as well.

There are amazing vaidyas even in present day India who can tell you your past and present ailments by just examining your pulse. There is one thing about pulse which I cannot rationalise– I do not forget the pulse of a patient even after a lapse of several years. I did not realise that until some people remarked when they came for consultation after a year or two and I told them about their pulse examination in comparison to what it was earlier. I am not a private practitioner and I concluded that since I examine very few persons every year, I could remember their pulse. However, after Vaidya Brahaspati Dev Triguna told me about one of his experiences with pulse, I am convinced that pulse examination is done at a profounder level by some vaidyas. Triguna ji used to see about 200 persons every day, thus he had very little time for each patient. When he felt the pulse of a person, his eyes were generally closed and he hardly looks at a person. He gives his diagnosis and prescribes a medicine. Once a woman patient was quite taken aback from his diagnosis and at the end of the day, she came to Triguna ji for the second time. After feeling her pulse, he said to her, 'You have already been here this morning?' The woman was embarrassed and extremely mystified. Her idea to come the second time was to be sure about her diagnosis and to testify the vaidya's mysterious ability to diagnose so quickly. The great vaidya even recognised her pulse despite having examined 200 odd pulses that day.

In modern India, there are two kinds of Ayurvedic education. There is a modern way by going to the university and the second is with guru-shishya tradition. This later education is more profound as compared to the classroom education because it is done with repeated practice and by gaining experience with a wise vaidya. For learning to do diagnosis with pulse, it is essential that one is associated with a master in this field and one is also persistent and concentrated. Concentration comes through yogic methods and imbibing sattva– the inner peace and stillness.

3

Methods of Pulse Diagnosis

Before concentrating on pulse diagnosis, it is important to know about the other diagnostic methods used in Ayurveda. For an Ayurvedic physician, the external appearance of a person is an indicator of his/her inner state of being. One observation indicates something and the physician follows it up with the other observations to confirm the diagnosis. For example, if a person has a pale skin, the physician will be apprehensive about the liver functions of this person. The examination of the tongue can confirm this diagnosis. Further questions about hunger, thirst, and stool lead to the finer analysis of the liver malfunctions. The pulse examination coordinates all the observations. A person's behaviour along with the pulse examination also reveals his/her psychic state and its influence on the body. That leads to the causative factors of the physical ailment if this is the case.

Since pulse examination is the principal theme here, after a brief description of the other diagnostic methods, I will go in details about the importance of pulse examination for a detailed diagnostics.

Ashtavidha Pariksha or the eightfold diagnosis

The eightfold examination that is generally used is the following:

1. Mala or the stool examination
2. Mutra or the urine examination
3. Jihva or the tongue examination
4. Shabda or the voice examination
5. Saparsha or the skin examination
6. Drika or the eye examination
7. Akriti or the examination of general appearance
8. Nadi or the pulse examination

Stool

Following are different diagnosis of stool:

- The healthy stool should be neither too hard and nor too soft in consistency and should be well formed.
- Dry and dark coloured stool in the shape of small balls speaks for vata vikriti.
- Stool of watery consistency and greenish colour denotes pitta vikriti.
- Sticky and whitish stool shows kapha vikriti.
- In case of vikriti of all the doshas, the stool is variable. Constipation followed by diarrhoea and slimy stool are the symptoms for vikriti of all the doshas.

102

Urine

Following are different diagnosis of urine:

- The healthy urine should be transparent and nearly like water.
- Turbid urine speaks for excess of air element in your body (vata).
- Yellow urine is indicative of too much heat in your body (pitta).
- If your urine has foam, it is because of the disturbance of water and earth element (kapha) in your body.
- If the urine becomes blackish in colour, that signifies the vikriti of all the doshas.
- The symptoms like difficulty in passing urine, or to get a burning sensation and accompanying pain when passing urine or slimy and turbid urine indicates some serious infection or disorder.

Tongue

Following are different diagnosis of tongue:
- A healthy tongue should be pink, clear and with lustre.
- A dry and rough tongue indicates vata vikriti.
- A feeling of burning, reddish in colour, with bitter taste and frequently growing blisters on the tongue are due to pitta vikriti.
- In kapha vikriti, the tongue gets white coating and it remains wet and slimy.

103

- If the above signs persists despite an effort to balance the doshas, that is indicative of a disorder in the system.

Voice examination

Following are different diagnosis of voice:
- In case of vata vikriti, a person sounds anxious and tends to speak very rapidly.
- In case of pitta vikriti, the voice may become cracked.
- In case of kapha vikriti, the voice may sound heavy or depressed in some cases, or the person may clear the throat frequently.
- Broken, low and weak voice with confusion in speech is indicative of vikriti of all the doshas and speaks for a disorder.

Skin examination

Quality of the skin along with the external body temperature should be examined by the physician. Here is the diagnosis of this examination:

- Rough, cold and dry skin is indicative of vata vikriti.
- Reddish, hot and oily skin with plenty of sweat is indicative of pitta vikriti. The sweat tends to smell bad.
- White, cold and moist skin is indicative of kapha vikriti.

- Cold hands and hot forehead, sudden feelings of hot and cold or bouts of sweat are indicative of imbalance of all the doshas or some specific disorders.
- Pale skin indicates disorders of agni or the digestive fire.

Eye examination

Following is the diagnosis for eyes:

- Dry and smoky appearance of the eyes is indicative of vata vikriti.
- Pink or red eyes and sensitivity to light (photophobia) is indicative of pitta vikriti.
- White and wet eyes are indicative of kapha vikriti.
- Lustreless and dull eyes are indicative of imbalance of all the doshas or some specific ailments.

Examination of general appearance

General appearance of the patient is observed in terms of their strength (*bala*), prakriti or any special feature besides the above described diagnostic methods. Bag under the eyes or a fatigued look or nervous and hectic behaviour or restless while sitting or listening to you are some of the very prominent features a physician should observe to find out prakriti and vikriti. The appearance of a person also shows whether he or she has an ailment and is suffering. Physician does this observation generally during the time when a patient is telling about his ailments or sufferings.

Pulse examination

Let us go into the details of this major diagnostic method, which is the principal theme here.

Before we proceed further with the pulse examination, it is important to clarify that Ayurveda is not only a system of medicine but it deals with life in general. It is integrated in everyday life of people as a way of life to enhance the quality of life. There are countless home remedies that people use to cure their minor ailments. The above-described diagnostic methods are not used exclusively by the physicians. Awareness about *mala* and about the general appearance of the body is a part of Ayurvedic awareness and forms commonsensical knowledge of many Indians for maintaining health. However, it is a physician (vaidya) who correlates various diagnostic methods and is able to go to the root cause of the ailment through medical wisdom. Pulse examination is a very important Ayurvedic diagnostic method for the vaidyas and is not a part of the home diagnostic methods like the ones described above. It is difficult as compared to the mala diagnostic methods and it needs proper training and an experience of several years.

Details of pulse examination

Subtlety in pulse examination

Pulse examination is the subtlest of all the diagnostic methods described above. In reality, all the Ayurvedic diagnosis is done at a very subtle level or in a yogic state. According to some Ayurvedic Acharyas, the diagnosis is a *sadhana* (accomplishment to achieve meditation) and one requires yogic power for it. Until the physician has a peaceful mental state and is completely concentrated during examination, it is not possible to understand the problems of the patient. The physician should examine with the combination of knowledge, experience and rationality. Besides that, the physician should be very friendly and compassionate. Sage Agnivesha in *Charaka Samhita* has told about one of the qualities of a physician is *sarvapranishu bandhubhuta*– a quality of universal brotherhood.

Yogic qualities like attention and concentration are specifically required for pulse examination. They help you to develop sensitivity which is very essential for pulse examination. I do not mean to say that the methods of pulse diagnosis are not based on *yukti* (rationality) as recommended by Charaka for all Ayurvedic diagnosis and medication. To distinguish between the fine notes of music you need fineness and sensitivity; similarly, you require that for pulse examination. I cite below few lines from Vaidya Gangasahaye Pande to make my idea more explicit.

107

The language and speech cannot express the feelings completely. With the change of tone, same word can have different meanings. ... The notes from Veena (an instrument like Sitar) evoke diverse feelings in people and it is not possible to express those feelings in words. Similarly, it is not possible to express in words the subtle variations in nature we observe with the sense of sight. The green colour of a parrot, of leaves of Ashoka tree, that of the paddy fields and of the leaves of lotus is different despite being green. The observer expresses himself/herself by using adjectives like bright, deep or light to describe the variations in the colour. Can the description like this convey the visualisation of the reality? .... It is the same situation with the pulse. Words can express the details of the pulse but there is a gap between the explanation and the ability to derive the conclusive results.[*]

In Ayurvedic literature, the pulse diagnosis is described in a very interesting manner by giving similes from the gait of different animals like snake, frog, peacock, duck, swan etc. To be able to learn from these similes from the ancient literature, you require a complete experience with nature. I have often heard student quote these similes that they have learnt with different Ayurvedic teachers without really feeling the profoundness of their meaning and

---

[*] Gangasahaye Pande, *Kayachikitsa (Hindi),* 1981, third edition, Chaukhambha Bharati Acadamy, Varanasi.

sense. I try to use different methods and similes so that modern people can relate better to them. It is appropriate to add here that it takes very long time and tremendous experience to get the ability to learn to do diagnosis through pulse examination.

Pulse diagnose can be compared to music. Music evokes certain feelings in a connoisseur whereas those who do not feel its subtlety, the fine nuances remain insensitive to it. Similarly, you have to gradually obtain mastery with practice and experience to be a connoisseur to understand the subtle variations in pulse in healthy persons of different prakriti, during the state of vikriti and during some major physical and mental disturbances in the body.

Rationality of pulse diagnosis in relation to vata, pitta and kapha

The three principal energies of the body or the doshas- vata, pitta and kapha work in coordination with each other. Let us understand the thermodynamics of the body with respect to the three doshas in order to comprehend the importance of pulse diagnosis. The three doshas work in coordination with each other and if any one of the doshas does not perform its one or more functions well, this affects also the other doshas. Let us take a very simple example. Pitta produces energy for the body. Energy comes from the digestion of the food we eat. For digestion, pitta needs digestive juices, which

109

are produced by kapha, as the formation of new cells and secretions are the function of kapha. Once the energy is produced, it should reach each and every part of the body. This is the function of vata to circulate this energy in the whole body and distribute it to each and every cell. The circulation of blood is the function of vata. Out of all the diagnostic methods, the blood circulation carries the most subtle and complete information on the body due to its access to each and every part of the body. Besides that, it carries the information on pitta and kapha as the energy the blood is carrying is the result of pitta and the quality of that energy depends upon the quality of kapha. That is because the secretions for the production of the pitta energy are formed by kapha. The rhythm of the flow of blood is indicated by the pulsation of the blood vessels. The pulsation varies in a very subtle manner according to the smoothness in the flow of blood. Smoothness of the flow of blood varies according to the energy it is using for flow (pitta) and the proportion of kapha in it.

When and how to feel the pulse

The best time to examine the pulse is early in the morning immediately after getting up but after relieving oneself. It is said that this time the pulse is not influenced by the activity of the doshas and the mind is at peace.

Pulse examination is done by putting three fingers on the wrist at the root of the thumb. In some texts, it is suggested that one should examine the left wrist in case of women and right wrist in case of men.

However, in the other texts this theory is discarded and stated that it does not really matter which wrist you use for the pulse examination. I personally agree with the latter view. The most important is that the person you are examining should be in a restful state and should be reclining. The physician should be also calm and concentrated. Pulse should not be examined after meals, after a hectic activity, after physical exercise or sexual intercourse. If someone has come from outside, give ten minutes of rest before you examine the pulse.

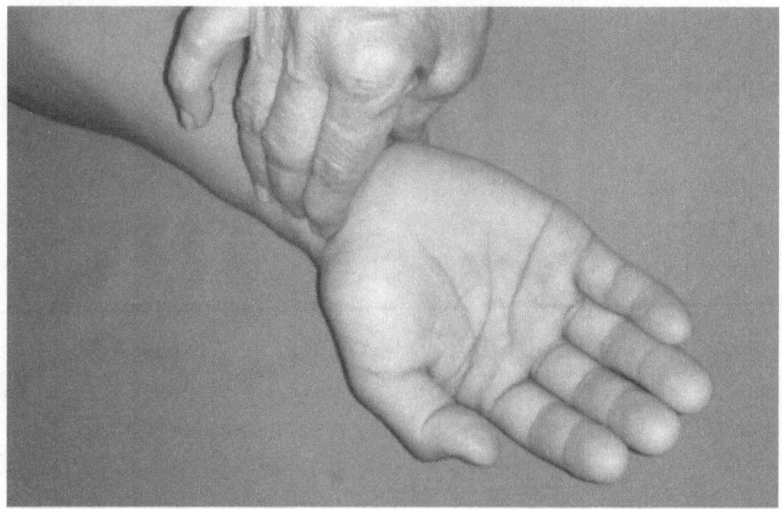

If you feel confused in some cases and find variability in the pulse, it is better to examine several times and after some rest, particularly early morning immediately after getting up.

A note about left and right pulse: There are exceptional vaidyas who see both left and right and they can diagnose the energy levels of two sides of the body. I have once a personal experience to this effect. I had broken the ligament of my left knee but it has healed in about six months. After a year from that, I had a distinguished opportunity to be examined Vaidya ... in Varanasi. He told me that despite the broken ligament, my left side had more energy and power than the right side. Over the years I realised how true the great Vaidya was. I also realised that since my left side had more power, I probably strained it more, thus leading to the tearing of the ligament.

Pulse and the individual variations

Ayurveda has become popular in Europe during the recent years. It seems like it is a very romantic and tender health science for the Westerns. Besides the tenderness of all its oil treatments and anointing, it leaves scope for individual variations and acceptance of that variation like you have seen in Part I of this book on Prakriti. People are not made to think that they are like machines and all of them should be similar and equally quick and rapid in their actions and reactions. It gives you your space and inner freedom to be different and to be able to assert that difference with dignity. Ayurveda lays a great emphasis on individual variations which is due to prakriti or the individual constitution. As has been already told in Part I, prakriti not only determines your physiological reactions but also your behavioural personality. It is like your inner face. There are as many variations in prakriti as we have different outward appearances in human beings. Variety and constant change are the essential factors of nature. Observe hundred plants and all of them have different shapes, form of leaves, colour of flowers, and so on. If we do not accept the variety in human beings, we are going against nature, which is an anti-health act.

For learning to examine pulse, you will have to take into account the individual variations and variability that exist in human beings. Diagnosis of vikriti and disorders is a far away step. It is not possible to learn diagnosis of ailments unless you are an expert in examining a normal and healthy pulse in all its musical variations.

For European lovers of Ayurveda, pulse examination is generally associated with prakriti. Many students in my weekend workshops think that they can learn *all* about pulse examination in short time. The long-term students in our school generally do not do enough practical homework to proceed further on this learning. I am narrating all this to emphasize that if you wish to learn about the pulse examination, you need long time for theory and practice. I give in the next chapter a programme in nine steps for about two years. To learn pulse examination properly is one of the hardest things in Ayurveda and there is no short cut to it. It is to learn to decode the codes the pulsation has, as its quality is the result of the journey of the blood in every part of the body. Before learning to decode the pulsation, you have to first learn to know their diversity. Thus, you need concentration, hard work and regular practice in order to learn the decoding of the pulsating blood vessels. It can be compared to sadhana (meditation). As you require ekagrata (concentration of the thought process on a single object) for sadhana, similarly you need that for learning the methods of diagnostics with pulse. It is a learning that requires repeated practice and persistence over a long period of time.

4

Nine-step method for learning pulse diagnosis

I have oriented this chapter in such a way that along with the theoretical description of the variations in the pulse of diverse persons and in the same person during different physiological and emotional states, the readers can also learn the practice of pulse examination. There is no doubt that one requires a practical experience with an able teacher to be a master of this diagnostic methods, nevertheless, the self-learning method below can give you a sound foundation. I have described this method in nine steps and over a period of two years.

Steps 1 to 5 are for three months each whereas steps 6 to 8 are done simultaneously in six months. Step nine is done for three months.

Step 1
Feeling the Pulse

Feel your own pulse: Feel exclusively your own pulse for three months, five to six times a day. Feel your pulse in diverse circumstances. Take care that you follow the above-described instructions about how to feel the pulse and collect the data. In the beginning, take the pulse at the following timings:

- In the morning, immediately after getting up.
- In the evening, shortly before sleeping. That means, after you have been lying in your bed for a brief period and are just going to sleep.
- During the day, take your pulse when you are:
  - hungry,
  - after meals,
  - tired,
  - feel good,
  - feel angry,
  - feel depressed.

Note down briefly each time the results of your examination. Write in your own way in the light of the knowledge you have obtained whatever comes to your mind or in whatever way you can express yourself. Be brief and write comparing the pulse of diverse examinations. For example, you may notice that your morning pulse one day was faster or louder than the other days. Note down that. Think of the reasons related to that and note them briefly as well. For example, 'my pulse was louder this morning than other days. It could be because I had a restless sleep or I drank too much tea or coffee the previous day or I was very thirsty during the night as I had a rather salty dinner in a restaurant, and so on'. Without any strain on your mind, write spontaneously the way you feel. You will realise that we all have some fundamental wisdom about our body but we are not attentive enough to interpret it. Your own frequent pulse examination will evoke this wisdom and you will not only learn a step in pulse examination but also have an experience of your inner being.

This training is to teach you to feel the diverse nuances of the pulse. It is your own body and you will learn to correlate the diverse phases you undergo during the day with the nadi sapandan (pulsation of the blood vessels). You will also learn about the effect of your emotions on your physiology.

Keep going through your notes from time to time and change the terminology in case you feel that you could express yourself in a better way.

After few weeks, you will gain confidence and then try to incorporate some other situations for pulse examination. Keep on your morning and evening routine, as that will enable you to distinguish the daily situation just like the other diagnostic practices of stool, urine, tongue, etc. Incorporate the the following in pulse examination for the second phase:
- After some concentration and meditative practices.
- After vigorous exercise like running or going up the stairs.
- In some special circumstances.

During the three months period, you may have some special circumstances like feeling very good due to some achievement or success or feeling disgusted of everything around you or having fever or pain or indigestion, etc. This will give you an opportunity to see another aspect of diversity of pulse diagnosis.

After this Step, you will acquire some sensitivity to hear various sounds and will begin to correlate them to the physiological and mental changes. You will get the training to distinguish the diversity in frequency, pitch, tonality and rhythm.

Step 2
Learn to interpret the data

Continue to feel your pulse another three months but this time, you try to interpret it with the knowledge about diverse types of pulsation your body's blood vessel undergo in different states and different circumstances.

First of all, it is essential to know the pulse for the three doshas. It does not however mean that it is for determining the prakriti of a person. It is in general and it could be related to the temporary phase the body is undergoing. For example, you may get the pitta results of the pulse during the process of digestion. Study carefully the following description and try to correlate it with the results you have obtained from your three months experience. Continue to take your pulse like you have been doing but interpreting your observations in the light of the information given below.

Pulse of a healthy person
- The pulse of a healthy person with balanced doshas is smooth, regular and softly strong. It is like the sound of a clock. It is smooth and regular tik..tik..tik..tik..tik.. The input and

output of the pulse is similar and pitch remains stable.

- The best time to obtain a well-balanced pulse of a healthy person is in the morning after getting up and after going to the toilet. At other times of the day, there may be some alterations.

- Pulse of a healthy person takes into account the prakriti of that person. Thus, the above description may be interspersed with slight alterations denoting the prakriti of a person.

Given below is the description of the pulse of three doshas. It is important to understand that in case you have equilibrium and have constant pulse like the description above, your pulse may also pulsate your dominant dosha or doshas from time to time depending upon the degree of domination. Thus, in a healthy and regular pulse, you will have alterations.

- Vata pulse is tik-tak...tik-tak...tik-tak...tik-tak...tik-tak. That means in the pulsation, the input is shorter and the output is longer. In Ayurvedic literature, vata pulse is compared to the gait of a leech or a snake.

- Pitta pulse is a jumpy pulse. The usual regular impulses are interspersed with sudden and fast impulses. Tik...tik...tik...tik...tik.tik.tik... In the Ayurvedic literature, it is described like the movements of a frog or a crow.

- Kapha pulse is a profound and relatively low in pitch as compared to the vata and pitta pulse. In other words, it is a heavy pulse. It is a pulse that is low and slow. It is like teek....teek...teek. It is described like the movements of a swan.

At this stage, another important fact to know is that the pulse of your dominating dosha is generally revealed intermittently in the healthy pulse but there are also some specific situations when the pulse signifies the other dosha. For example, when you are hungry, your pulse may be unstable and feeble. After having eaten, it will become stronger and stable again. However, during the first hour of digestion, you may get some signs of pitta pulse. If you do walking or some other physical work, pulsation is more likely to alter to pitta pulsation.

This step is complicated as compared to the first one as in the first step, you were just learning to listen. The most important in the first step was to get used to the difference in pitch, intensity and rhythm. In this step, there is recognition of all that and the interpretation of their meaning. You will realise that with the repeated practice for three months, you would develop sensitivity to diversity.

Step 3
Pulse in diverse circumstances

This step comprises of creating different circumstances to measure the pulse in order to feel the pulsation in diverse conditions. For the next three months, take the data on your pulse in the following special situations:

- After a vigorous exercise like running or jumping or bicycling very fast.
- After an oil massage.
- After svedana (fomentation or sweat therapy).
- After yogasanas.
- After japa or any other form of meditative practices.

I give below in the boxes the home method for doing oil massage and fomentation on your own.

Oil saturating self-massage

- Choose a warm corner of your house if it is cold weather. Take some warm oil and start applying with your right hand on your left hand. After applying on each finger and on both sides of your hand, massage the hand with pressure. Massage individually each finger.
- Apply the oil on whole arm in long and strong stokes. Apply oil also on your shoulder and underarm. Go on massaging so that the oil gets absorbed. Keep applying more oil if needed. Different people need different quantity of oil depending upon their prakriti or state of vikriti.
- Repeat the same with your left hand on your right hand and arm.
- Massage with plenty of oil your left foot. Use both your hands. Apply oil on the lower leg with long stokes and applying good pressure so that the oil is absorbed. Similarly massage

---

> the whole leg and subsequently repeat the same on right foot and leg.
>
> - Stand up and apply oil on your buttocks and both the sides of your torso. Apply pressure to get the oil absorbed.
> - Sit down again and apply oil on front part of your body, neck and face by the application of oil and massage strokes several times.
> - Apply oil on your lower back by extending your arms behind and on upper back by taking your arms from above. In case you have problems, take a plastic sheet, smear oil on it and role with your back on it
> - To saturate the body completely, repeat the whole process two more times.

It is advisable to take the wet fomentation after the oil massage.

Wet fomentation

In Ayurveda, fomentation or perspiration therapy is of two kinds- dry and wet. Dry consists of sweating in dry and hot place (like a sauna) and wet is like a vapour bath. However, in Ayurveda, exposing to cold or air is strictly forbidden after fomentation therapy. I describe below a simple method to do wet fomentation at home done in a bathtub.

- Before your bath, make sure that you close all the windows and the place should be warm. Prepare your bed and make it warm with a hot water bottle. Make some ginger + basil + cardamom + pepper tea in a thermos and keep it besides your bed.

- Prepare a hot bath. Add some drops of essential oils like rose, jasmine, fennel or their combination into it. Sit in the bath comfortably and make sure that the water remains hot. Add more hot water from time to time.
- When you start sweating, come out of your bath, put on a bathrobe and go to your warm bed. Take some tea and rest fully covered in the bed. You will continue to sweat for a while.
- Rest for about ½ an hour after you have stopped sweating.

This step is for teaching you the variations in the quality of the pulse in various circumstances. You get a jumpy and excited pulse after a vigorous exercise whereas a quieter pulse after various anti-stress and relaxed measures like massage and fomentation.

In this step, you are observing the diversity from the normal pulse. Note the differences in the above-described circumstances.

- After a vigorous exercise, the pulse is very fast and loud. You will realise that after about 30 seconds, the pulse begins to calm down. The rhythm becomes slower and pitch becomes lower. During youth, this reversal to normal is faster whereas aging prolongs this time.
- After oil massage and a little rest thereafter, pulse is generally calm and regular.
- After fomentation, pulse is low and weak. Take a hot drink after fomentation and measure the pulse again. You will realise that it becomes louder and stronger within few minutes.

123

- After yogic exercises and a little rest with postures like shava asana or the dead body posture, the pulse is regular and strong.
- After japa or any kind of meditative practice, the pulse is strong but its duration is longer.

During this period, begin to feel the pulse of people in your immediate surroundings. Since you cannot have special circumstances all the time, take advantage of feeling the pulse of persons in your immediate surroundings. It will be beneficial to take the pulse of the same individuals at least three times a day. Compare your own pulse to the pulse of other persons taken in the similar circumstances. Next step is devoted entirely on this theme.

Step 4

Pulse examination of diverse individuals

For three months, take the pulse of diverse individuals. Your case study should be limited to healthy individuals. During this time, feel the pulse of as many persons as you can and in diverse circumstances. Make notes of diversity that you come across. If you feel that some individual have a pulse which does not fit in your knowledge obtained until now, make notes of this data with a question mark. May be you will get your answers as we proceed further.

During this step, incorporate different age groups and collect some data on different circumstances in these cases. It is not all that easy but at least do the data on different individuals after vigorous exercise and after meditation and observe carefully the difference obtained on the persons of different age groups.

The data of this step may be confusing for you at times as now you are exposed to diversity and you may come across several persons with vikriti. This step is an exposure to the diversity that can exist with the combination of age and circumstances. This step prepares you for the next step where you will learn about pulse in the state of vikriti.

Step 5
Pulse in the state of vikriti

This step involves taking pulse of the individuals who are tired, nervous, hectic (vata vikriti), easily angry (pitta vikriti), drowsy or lethargic (kapha vikriti). As is evident from the description of the fundamentals of Ayurveda, these are the individuals with vikriti of the doshas. Try to find more features for vikriti with the help of the descriptions given earlier in Chapter 1. Try not to take individuals in your study who are forever complaining of some health problems. These are generally the cases who have vikriti of one dosha for a long time and that has led to the vikriti of the other doshas as well. This kind of pulse will be confusing for you at this stage.

This step should also be for three months.

Here is the description of the pulse during dosha vikriti.

- In case of vata vikriti, the pulse is tik...tak...tik...tak...tik...tak. When a person of vata vikriti is made to rest and relax for a while, it is quite possible that the pulse comes back to normal, at least partially. This however, depends upon the extent of vikriti.
- A jumpy pulse denotes pitta vikriti. Tik... tik...tik...tik.tik.tik.tik. In between there are rapid and sudden pulsations. They are repeated at certain intervals.
- A kapha vikriti pulse is very low and heavy and dragging. Imagine the way you walk when you are carrying lot of weight on yourself. You feel the pulsation as if it is coming from a faraway place.

Step 6, 7 and 8
Vata vikriti
Pitta vikriti
Kapha vikriti

These three steps will be done in six months. I have put them together for convenience, as you will find diverse case studies at random. Who so ever you find, you will have to classify according to their vikriti. Secondly, these three steps together are meant to train you in two more things than what you learnt already in step 5.

- The pulse of a dosha vikriti can be variable and that denotes the extent and specificity of the vikriti. For example a vata vikriti person may be nervous, or have disturbed sleep or is constipated. These facts can be differentiated from the pulse.
- Mixed vikriti of two doshas is another feature that has to be taken into consideration at this stage.

Variations in pulse due to diverse symptoms of vata vikriti

Emotions and worries: A person with vata vikriti is excessively emotional, worries a lot and is easily fearful. Under emotional pressure or due to fear, there are certain vibrations on the descending pulse. Ascending pulse is slightly louder but descending pulse has a vibrating echo.

Insomnia: Vata vikriti can also have sleep disturbances and insomnia. In these conditions, pulse is rather hectic but with a gap. The time of pulsation of up and down is very fast but there is a larger gap between the two pulsations.

Dry skin, dry throat and constipation are other features of vata vikriti. This is the case of vata vitiation when one feels dried out in the body. The pulsation has less force and the descending pulse is shorter than the ascending pulse.

Variations in pulse due to diverse symptoms of pitta vikriti

Long and difficult digestion: The principal vikriti of pitta is that of the disturbance of agni or digestive fire. The pulsation suddenly changes in duration, pitch and frequency. The regular pulse changes into shorter and sudden pulsations. During the process of digestion, the pulse is lower in pitch also when it has a regular duration.

Excessive hunger and thirst: The pulse is very restless and changes in rhythm. Before meal times, the pulsation becomes short in duration very frequently. This state gets back to normal after hunger and thirst is appeased.

Easily angry and feeling excessively heat: Pulse in this case of pitta vikriti is loud and high in frequency and suddenly breaks down in very short impulses. However after some cooling treatment or change of weather or calming down after a bout of anger, the pulse stabilises.

Variations in pulse due to diverse symptoms of kapha vikriti

Excessive sleep and drowsiness: The pulse is very low and heavy as if somebody is going through a passage with difficulty. The pitch is very low as well.

Cold and wet hands and feet: The pulse is slower than the above mentioned and has lesser frequency and pitch in comparison.

Tendency to build phlegm: In this case of kapha vikriti, pulse sounds very dull and low in frequency. The time of ascend and descend of the pulsation is longer than the above described two situations.

Vikriti of two doshas

It is quite possible to get confused in some cases, especially when a person has vikriti of more than one dosha. This is where you need your complete concentration and previously obtained knowledge. For example, if you see a pulse with vata vikriti that goes tik-tak-tik-tak and so on but it has a vibration during tak or the descending pulsation. That makes you conclude that the person has vata vikriti and some worries or specific fear. In other words, there is emotional instability and insecurity. While you are observing this pulse and driving all these conclusions, you suddenly feel that the pulse is varying suddenly and sounding tik.tik.tik.. in a jumping manner. Obviously, the person has vata and

129

pitta vikriti simultaneously. In this situation, you have to also take care that you are not taking the pulse when the person is hungry. In case of any doubt, repeat the pulse examination empty stomach in the morning hours.

Similarly, you can have vata-kapha and kapha-pitta vikriti. From a careful examination of the pulse, you can also distinguish the degree of the vitiation of two doshas and the specific ailments they are causing.

It is important that you validate your results by asking your subjects other questions. Thus, for learning well the pulse examination, you should have the fundamental wisdom of Ayurveda regarding the dynamic aspects of prakriti and vikriti.

Step 9
Vikriti of all the doshas

When all the doshas are in a state of vikriti, the body functions get gradually out of balance. In the state of health, doshas accumulate energy for performing body functions in the form of *dhatus*. Dhatus are seven in number and they provide support and nourishment to the body. In case of vikriti of all the doshas, the dhatus are no more nourished. Dhatus are a supporting system of the body and they deplete in these conditions. Weakness and disease follow if this occurs.

The difficult situation for pulse examination is when you find almost everything you have learnt until now in the pulse of one individual. You may get only very few subjects who have vikriti of all the doshas. In fact, these persons have already an ailment or a disorder or they are standing at the threshold of being ill. Such persons need immediate help to revert back to normalcy. They need a change of diet, and lifestyle, and medication to come back to more or less normal conditions. After this initial treatment, they should be given rasayanas to promote their vitality and immunity. After this initial treatment, they would ultimately need complete panchakarma in order to uproot the imbalance. It is said in Ayurveda that curing imbalance with medications is like cutting a tree from its stem. In this case, the tree is still not dead and it gives rise to offshoots. However, with panchakarma treatment, the imbalances are completely uprooted.

To understand the pulse examination for complicated cases where you find imbalance of all the doshas, it is important that you understand profoundly the interrelationship of the doshas with each other. If vata is imbalanced, there is a lack of kapha as well. The light element without the absence of a heavy element is more light and its movements are faster. For example, to control a hectic state of mind (excess of element akasha or the space), you need more of the earthy element to balance it. Similarly, if kapha is excessive, the fire element can balance it. It is cold and wet and with heat, it comes to balance. The excess of fire element is balanced with the earth and water elements. Imbalance of vata makes the fire go up and down thus causing its imbalance as well. One imbalance leads to another and thus ultimately the whole system becomes disorganised.

Pulse in this state of vikriti and depletion of dhatus is altering very often. It shifts from vata vikriti pulse to pitta or kapha and again back. If the duration of the vikriti has been very long and there is considerable depletion of the dhatus (*dhatukshaya*), the pulse sounds also very low and lacking any force. But the alterations are still there from one vikriti to another. You will realise that the shift is quite sudden and one kind of vikriti pulse is variable in its duration.

After doing the practice of pulse examination for two years and in nine steps, you will get used to the tremendous variety of rhythm, tonality, pitch and strength that you would be able to feel the pulsating blood vessel and the extraordinary information this pulsation carries.

Described below are some other factors you need to pay attention to.

Relationship of pulse to age

Children have a very soft pulse but it is regular in healthy state and it has 'lubricating movements'. The pulsation is shorter in duration. That means the consistency of the fluid (blood) is smooth and with appropriate fat contents. However, the pitch and vigour of the pulse is variable during childhood depending upon prakriti or state of vikriti.

During youth, pulse is loud with long duration and sharp pitch. Long duration of pulse means longer than the childhood. In fact, in Sanskrit, this pulse is called 'pooran' that means complete or full.

The pulse of old persons is slow, deep, dry and at times hindered. This terminology needs some explanation. Quite contrary to the pulse of a child, the pulse of an old person gives you the impression of being 'dry', meaning thereby that the consistency of the liquid flowing is lacking in lubrication and smoothness. Deep means with a profound sound and longer pulsation time. Slow signifies the frequency.

The pulse of a pregnant woman is heavy and slow. The pitch is lower in the beginning of ascending pulse whereas it is louder towards the end.

Relationship of pulse to lifespan

I have described earlier the pulse of a healthy person. There are some subtle variations in the healthy pulse that denote the lifespan of a person. A healthy pulse which is very forceful and smooth and very precisely regular denotes a very strong fundamental constitution, high ojas (immunity and vitality) and long life. A regular pulse but with less force and strength speaks for a medium long lifespan. If despite being extremely regular, the pulse sounds like a slow flowing river, it is signifies relatively low ojas and an average or below average lifespan.

Prakriti and Pulse in Ayurveda (Pulse)

The important factor in this description is the correlation of the effort we make to safeguard our health and the health we have from our birth. In Ayurveda, *daiva* is what we bring with us at birth from our previous karma and *purushkara* is what we do with the karma or our deeds of this life. For good health and longevity, one needs to coordinate between one's daiva and purushkara. Our purushkara should be in such a way that we do our best with the state of health we have brought with us from birth. If born with good health, the effort should be to preserve it and if there are some problems, one should find all ways and means to improve the existing conditions and then enhancing the ojas or the basic energy level. If someone has a pulsation that speaks for longevity but this person does not take care of his/her health or do deeds that are anti-health, the lifespan will be reduced. Similarly the person with a medium or average lifespan can have longer life if he or she does purification practices, take rasayanas (ojas-promoting substances) and leads an Ayurvedic lifestyle according to desha (place) and kala (time– of the day, year, one's age).

5

Pulse in pathological conditions

According to Ayurveda, diseases are three kinds—endogenous, exogenous and psychic. Endogenous diseases are those which arise due to a long-term imbalance of the doshas. These originate due to an erred lifestyle and neglect for oneself. Blood pressure, allergies, haemorrhoids, arthritis, sleep disturbances are some examples of this category. Exogenous disorders are due to external infections of parasites or poisons. Psychic ailments are due to not getting what one desires or forced to live with the undesired.

In the previous chapter, I have described the pulse examination during the state of vikriti. When the state of vikriti of one dosha is left unattended, it enhances and ultimately it disturbs the balance of the other two doshas as well. When one of the three energies is sluggish or disturbed, obviously, the whole system gets disturbed thereby giving rise to a disorder in the long run. Thus, when one has vikriti of more than one dosha, one is already standing at the threshold of a disorder. If the vikriti is left unattended for a long time, one falls prey to one or more endogenous ailments. As described in the previous chapter, the dhatus deplete in this condition and the ojas of the body (immunity and vitality) go down in the state of vikriti of all the doshas. Thus, one becomes vulnerable to exogenous disorders as well. When the body is unwell and weak and one is suffering from ailments, one tends to become mentally down and becomes susceptible to psychological ailments as well. Thus, from the holistic point of view of Ayurveda, everything is interconnected, interrelated and interdependent.

During certain endogenous ailments, pulse is more intense and distorted form of the vikriti pulse. In serious and chronic disorders, pulse is very erratic and in each case you need to examine many persons over a long period of time to get mastery for doing correct diagnosis by examining the pulse. All the descriptions of pulse examination up to vikriti are not valid in such cases. Pulse has variations depending upon the complexity of the disorder. Given below are the descriptions of the pulse during some common ailments and disorders.

Fever

There are three kinds of fevers in Ayurveda according to three doshas. The vata fever pulse is like vata vitiation but very loud and fast. Although the fever is from vata disturbance, but heat by itself is a characteristics of pitta. Pulse is very fast and loud during pitta fever but it is jumpy intermittently. Kapha fever has low pulse but becomes very loud with short intervals. After a while, when the fever is slightly down, the pulsation becomes depressed in pitch again.

Diarrhoea

There are persons who suffer from excessive intestinal motility without any external infection. They go to the toilet several times and the quantity of mala (excrement) is excessive and assimilation of food (rasa) is low. This ailment is called *grahani* in Ayurveda. The pulse in case of grahani is loud with vibrations. It is forceful for certain duration whereas it feels weak sporadically.

In case of severe diarrhoea due to a bacterial or viral infection or due to the intake of some poisonous substances, the pulse is loud and vibrating during the ascending pulsation while the descending pulse has a shriller pitch.

Hypertension or high blood pressure

In case of hypertension, the pulse is very loud. It can be compared to the sound of a drum that is piercing loud. In fever, it is loud but does not resonate. In high blood pressure, the pulse makes a kind of echo.

Hypo tension or low blood pressure

Contrary to the above situation, in case of below normal blood pressure, the pulse has much less force and sounds kind of depressed and far away. The pulse rate is also lower.

Arthritis

The pulse is of vata vitiation and in between becomes very low with signs of kapha vitiation. In case the ailment is advanced, the pulse becomes very low and irregular. But it changes in volume from time to time.

Haemorrhoids or piles

In case of haemorrhoids, the pulse is extreme vata vitiation, loud and unstable. When the ailment is old, the pulse also shows the signs of pitta vitiation. It changes from slow to fast impulses.

Skin ailments

In skin ailments, the pulse sounds very hard and short. There is a lack of *snehan* or the fat element, which is responsible for the smoothness of the pulse.

Urinary ailments

In case of urinary ailments, pulse is very heavy and prolonged. In mild infection, it may seem to have normal volume but in acute cases, it sounds very low and weak.

Obesity

Sometimes it is difficult to find the pulse of over-weight and obese persons as the pulse is very low and they have lot of adipose tissue. The pulse of such persons is heavy, tired and low. It is like somebody is walking with a great effort.

Arrhythmia

The pulsation of the blood vessels denotes heartbeat. Arrhythmia is a pathological condition which is said to be in common language as 'heart missing a beat'. It is a disorder of the normal beating of the heart. It could be due to over exhaustion, use of drugs or some kind of disorder in sinus node, the normal cardiac pace maker.

It is easy to detect this disorder from the pulse. Occasional arrhythmia can be from fatigue and is corrected with appropriate rest and diet. However, if arrhythmia persists, it can affect the functions of the heart. Therefore, by simple method of controlling your pulse regularly, you can attend to this problem immediately.

Pulse in arrhythmia has uneven pulsations. Some pulsations are with great force whereas immediately after, there is pulsation of extremely low pitch and sound. There may be one or more pulsations like that and again, there will be some forceful pulsations.

Diabetes

The pulse of a diabetic person in the beginning of the ailment is regular but is little shrill. If the ailment persists and it is not treated, the pulse becomes weak and shriller. At the same time, it shows signs of vata vikriti. Thus, when the disease is at its peak, the pulse is low in volume, has sign of vata vikriti and sounds shrill.

Chronic cough and asthma

In these ailments pulse is low with small impulses but regular and stable when there is no attack. During attack, the pulse is very rapid and loud and intermittently irregular. It goes loud to low at intervals.

Insomnia and sleep disorders

In this ailment, the pulse is extreme vata vikriti pulse. There is tik-tak but this is longer in duration and at times there is a little gap between tik and tak. In case these disorders are caused due to excessive worry or fear, there is a vibration in the pulse along with the above pattern.

Diverse emotional problems

Short-term state of emotional imbalance translates into vikriti pulsation whereas a long-term state of emotional disturbance is considered like a malady. Here is the description of pulse in some emotional states.

Perpetual anger and dissatisfaction: Pulse of a person with these symptoms is a pitta vikriti pulse in an extreme manner. That means there are long durations of hopping pulsation shorter durations of normal pulsation.

Perpetual anxiety and worry: There are persons who are constantly anxious about events of life or day-to-day happenings. Their pulse is an extreme vata pulse along with vibrations in pulsation. For example the pulse of these subjects is a long tik...tak...tik...tak...tik..., and pulsation has vibrations. In case of excessively anxious persons, the pulsation is also loud.

Sad and depressed mental state: The pulse of these individuals is like extreme kapha vikriti pulse but it is even more lowly sounding and slower. The duration of each pulsation seem to linger on and than with a slight gap, there is a slow and prolonged descend.

Mental disturbances

In case of extreme mental disturbances when the patient has lost most of his/her rationality and coordination, the pulse is fast and loud and then suddenly becomes very low and sinking. It recovers back again to high volume. Thus, in this case, when the pulse is low, the physician should not think that patient is going to coma or is suffering from an incurable disorder.

Shock, fainting or excessive weight lifting

Some people may faint when they suffer from a shock. Shock could be due to falling from some height or otherwise in case of an accident, or after hearing a bad news. In fact, in both the cases the shock is mental as also in case of an accident, it is the fear of death that plays an important part to bring the person in an unconscious state. There are other persons who may faint after carrying excessive weight or due to working more than their capacity.

In case of fainting due to whatever reason, the pulsation is low to such an extent that it is very hard to find it. In some cases, pulsation may also disappear for a brief period. One should massage hands and feet of the person so that the pulsation recovers.

Pulse of a serious ailment

When the pulse is slipping away from under your fingers and sometimes you feel it very low under the other finger than you were first feeling, it signifies a serious ailment and the patient needs an immediate treatment. The pulse also becomes low and high very often and changes its pitch as well. However, this pulse should not be confused with the pulse of an incurable ailment.

142

Prananashini pulse (Pulse indicating death)

In Sharngadhara Samhita, there is a description of a pulse that is indicator of death (III, 5) and it is called prananashini pulse. Prana means the living element inside us. Body and soul stay together and their connection is nourished with constant breathing. Breathing is the cosmic link of an individual. When the breathing stops, life ends. That is why the inhalation and exhalation of the vital air is also called prana. Nashini means destructive.

Prananashini pulse is low and without any force. Thus, the flow of the blood is very low. Besides that after about 20-25 seconds of pulsation, there is a gap of 2 to 4 seconds. Again there is pulsation for about 20 seconds and that is followed by a gap of few seconds. The pulsation and the gap without pulsation is constantly repeated with the same rhythm. This pulse is an indicator of the end of life.

Doot nadi vigyan (Science of pulse of the messengers)

I have mentioned in the earlier part of this section of the book that pulse examination needs sattva– the stillness and peace of mind and it is done at a higher state of consciousness. In Ayurveda, it is said that a good physician can know the state of the patient by examining the patient's messenger. There is a whole body of literature with the above-mentioned name that prescribes the pulse examination of the messenger to know the state of the patient. With no personal experience in this field, I will not vouch for its validity. In my private sessions, sometimes people talk about their immediate family members and ask me some remedies for a particular ailment. From their brief description, mostly the prakriti of the unseen person is clear to me. But I will not see the pulse of another person who is a medium for the sick person. In Charaka Samhita, it is advised to work with *yukti* or rationality. Thus, personally I find an element of fantasy in the 'Doot nadi Vigyan'. Nevertheless, I think it is important for you to know about it as it is much talked about subject when it comes to the subject of pulse examination.

CONCLUSION

The reader should keep in mind that pulse diagnosis is one of the several Ayurvedic diagnostic methods and is not meant to be taken independently of the other methods of diagnosis. Although I have given examples of some exclusive vaidyas who can tell you a lot merely with pulse examination, but these are rare persons or sages and not everybody has the capability to do that. Therefore I suggest to the readers that they should learn the pulse diagnosis but they should validate their results with the help of other diagnostic methods as well.

In the chapter on the pulse in pathological conditions, I have limited myself to some selective ailments. This is a very broad theme and the purpose of this book is to address the general reader and trainees of these oriental schools of medicines all over the world. These enthusiasts of the oriental wisdom are very rarely doctors and only few of them are even paramedics. In any case, this section on Ayurvedic pulse diagnosis is to initiate you into learning the world of sound in our inner being in its variety and rhythm. Even if you are not interested in application of this diagnosis on others, the methods described here can help you to know yourself better.

This description of pulse diagnosis can provide a new and modern way to learn pulse diagnosis for the students of Ayurvedic medicine in India. You can begin its practice independently early enough in order to become an expert by the time you complete your degree and begin practicing. The classroom education does not always provide this kind of independent plans and programmes to learn. Once you get initiated in this practice through the pages of this section, you can further advance your knowledge by working with a good vaidya.

Pulse diagnosis is a simple and costless diagnostic method and can help you obtain the knowledge about your own body. By persistently feeling your pulse, you will also develop some intuitive wisdom for your inner world. I believe that no doctor in the world or diagnostic techniques can know your ailments and problems better than you yourself. Pulse examination is a simple way to know yourself better.

OM SHANTI

About the Author

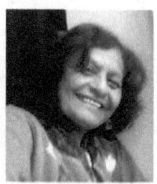 Along with a doctorate degree in reproduction biology in India, Dr. Verma studied Neurobiology in Paris University and obtained a second doctorate. She pursued advanced research at the National Institutes of Health, Bethesda (USA) and the Max-Planck Institute in Freiburg, Germany. At the peak of her career in medical research in a pharmaceutical company in Germany, she realised that the modern approach to health care is basically fragmented and non-holistic. Besides, we are directing all our efforts and resources to cure disease rather than maintaining health. In response, Dr. Verma founded The New Way Health Organisation (NOW) in 1986 to spread the message of holistic living, preventive methods for health care and to promote the use of mild medicine and various self-help therapeutic measures.

Dr. Verma grew up with a strong familial tradition of Ayurveda with a grandmother who had enormous Ayurvedic wisdom and was a gifted healer. She has studied Ayurveda in the traditional Guru-shishya style with Acharya Priya Vrat Sharma of the Benares Hindu University for 23 years.

Dr. Verma is an ardent researcher and is working hard to compile the living tradition of Ayurveda and spread it in the world through her books and other activities. She has published twenty three books on yoga, Ayurveda, Women and Companionship. The books are published in various languages of the world. Besides, she has published numerous scientific articles. Several other books are in preparation. She lectures extensively, teaches in Europe for several months a year, trains students at her two centres in India and gives radio and television programmes. A film on Ayurveda with her was made by German television in 1995 and was shown in 100 countries, in 130 languages. It was the first film on Ayurveda.

Dr. Verma has founded Charaka School of Ayurveda to train interested people with genuine Ayurvedic education so that they can further impart the knowledge of Ayurvedic way of life and save people from becoming a victim of charlatanry in Ayurveda. She is doing several research projects on medicinal plants and their combination in the form of remedies. She is the founder and chairperson of *The Ayurveda Health Organisation*, which is a charitable trust for distributing and promoting

Prakriti and Pulse in Ayurveda

Ayurvedic remedies and yoga therapy in rural areas of India. She does regular lectures and workshops for school children in the rural and remote areas of the Himalayas to promote wisdom of traditional science and medicine. Dr. Verma gives seminars, lectures and teaches in the *Charaka School of Ayurveda* with guru-shishya tradition.

For more information and contacts for Dr. Verma's school and teaching programme see www.ayurvedavv.com and www.drvinodverma.com

Dr. Vinod Verma's Publications

1. *Patanjali's Yoga Sutra: A Scientific Exposition* (Published in English, Hindi and German).

2. *Ayurveda for Inner Harmony: Nutrition, Sexual Energy and Healing* (Published in English, German, Italian, French, Romanian and Hindi).

3. *Ayurveda a Way of Life* (Published in English, German, Italian, French, Spanish, Czech, Greek, Portuguese, Slovenian and Hindi).

4. *The Kamasutra for Women* (Published in English [America and India], German, French, Dutch, Romanian, Italian, Portuguese, Slovenian Hindi and Malayalam).

5. *Stress-free Work with Yoga and Ayurveda* (Published in German, English [America and India] and Hindi).

6. *Patanjali and Ayurvedic Yoga* (Published in English, German and Hindi).

7. *Programming Your Life with Ayurveda* (Published in German, French, English, Slovenian and Czech).

8. *Ayurvedic Food Culture and Recipes* (Published in English, German, Czech and Hindi).

9. *Yoga: A Natural Way of Being* (Published in English, German, French, Italian and Hindi).

10. *Companionship and Sexuality: Based on Ayurveda and the Hindu tradition* (Published in English and German).

11. *Natural Glamour: The Ayurveda Beauty Book* (Published in German, Spanish and English)

12. *Losing and Maintaining Weight with Ayurveda and Yoga* (Published in English, Slovenian and German).

13. *The Timeless Wisdom of Ayurveda: A Scientific Exposition* (Published in English and German)

14. *Prakriti and Pulse: The Two Mysteries of Ayurveda* (Published in English)

15. *Good Food for Dogs: Vegetarian nourishment based on Ayurvedic wisdom* (Published in German and English)

16. *Diet for Losing Weight* (published in German and English)

17. *Aum: The Eternal Energy* (Published in German and English)

18. *Pulse Diagnose in Chinese and Ayurvedic Medicine* (co-author for TCM Dr. Florian Ploberger) (published in German)

19. *Shiva's Secrets for Health and Longevity* (published in German and English)

20. *Healing Hands: The Ayurvedic Massage workbook* (published in English)

21. *Prevention of Dementia* (published in German and English)

22. *Ayurveda for Dogs* (published in German and English)

23. Numerology: Based on the Vedic Tradition (published in English and Slovenian)

The Charaka School of Ayurveda and Patanjali Yogadarshana Society (Himalayan Centre)

The Charka School of Ayurveda (CSA) has been founded by Dr. Vinod Verma to spread the genuine classical tradition as well as the living tradition of Ayurveda in the world for promoting healthy living and preventing ailments. Its aim is to teach people a healthy lifestyle which enhances immunity and vitality and enables them to live a life with an optimum level of energy. For minor ailments, people should be capable of using home remedies, appropriate physical and mental exercises and nutrition.

CSA aims to bring genuine and practical aspects of Ayurveda to people and save them from Americanised and Europeanised distorted versions of Ayurveda and other forms of charlatanry that do more harm than good.

To achieve this purpose, CSA organises to train students in Europe who can further spread the message of Ayurvedic lifestyle and help people with genuine massages, purification practices, nutrition and other practical aspects of Ayurveda. The school is in association with the most learned persons of Ayurveda in India and several exclusive persons involved in health education in Europe.

The object of Patanjali Yogadarshana Society is to spread the message of Patanjali in the world. The wisdom of the Yoga Sutras is not only beneficial for the yogis but also for our day-to-day normal life. Its aim is to enhance *sattva* or the inner stillness and peace in the world as well as in the individual minds. With years of research on Yoga and Ayurveda, Dr. Verma has founded the Ayurvedic Yoga and has written a book on the subject.

Lectures, Seminars and Training Programmes

To get detailed information on the Charaka School of Ayurveda as well as our other programmes in India and Europe, visit our website or contact us by email.

The New Way Health Organisation .NOW.

A-130, Sector 26, Noida 201301, U.P., India
Tel. 0091 (0)120 2527820 or (0) 9873704205 or (0)9412224820
www.ayurvedavv.com www.drvinodverma.com
Contact at: ayurvedavv@yahoo.com

Prakriti and Pulse in Ayurveda (Pulse)

Himalayan Centre

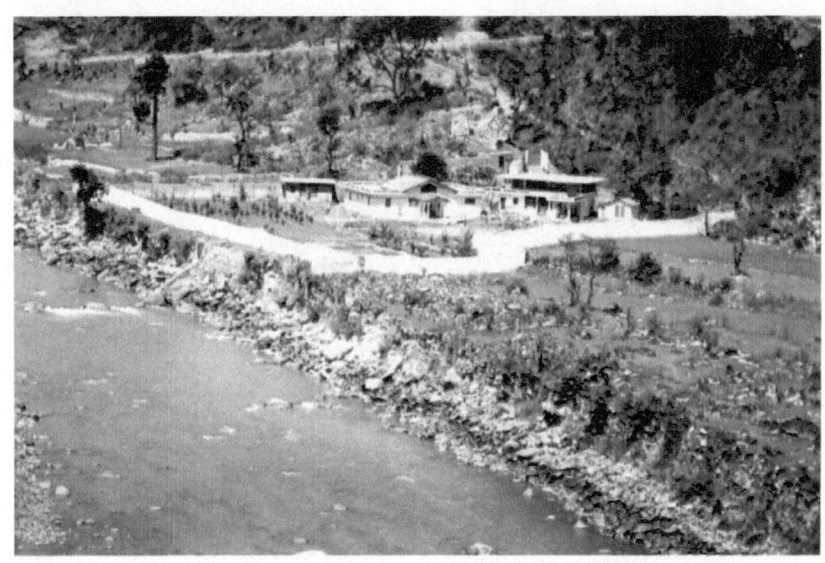

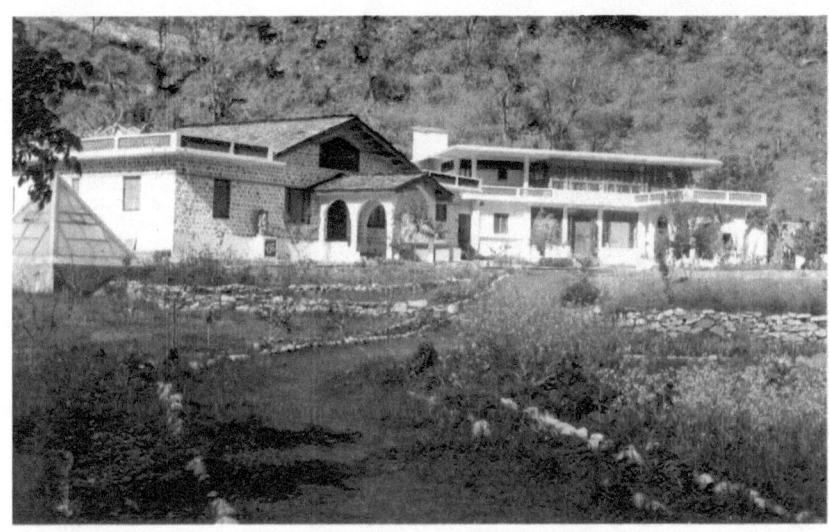

Companionship and Sexuality in Ayurveda and the Hindu Tradition

This book is not available in the market any more. We have some limited edition in four colours and can be directly ordered with us. The book costs 39 $. For a special price, (29 $ including postage) please write to Vanaja Vishal at ayurvedavv@gmail.com.

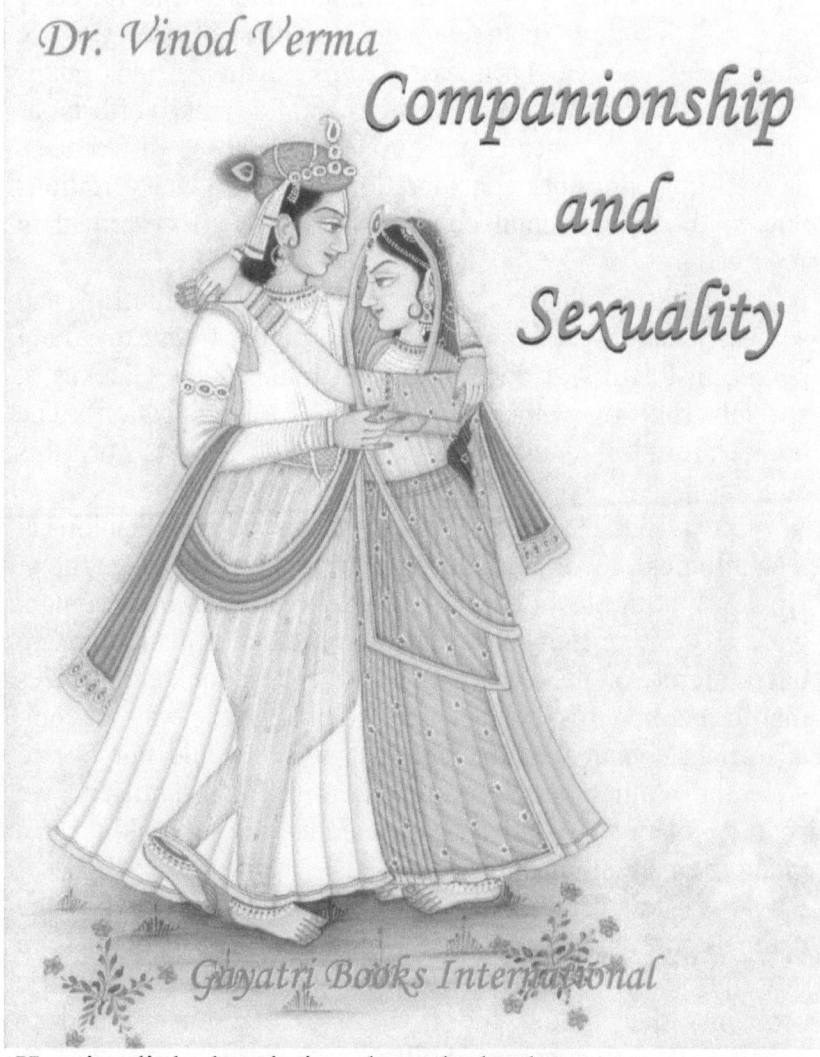

Here is a little description about the book.

Companionship and Sexuality

Sexuality is considered holy in the Hindu tradition and intense sexual experience leads to the cosmic bliss. One of the eight disciplines of medicine in Ayurveda is devoted to sexuality and rejuvenation. Sexuality is also considered as the basis of existence in terms of cosmic continuity in Ayurveda, as well as in other scriptures of the Hindu tradition. Based on this tradition, the author has analysed the primordial differences between men and women due to the different ratio of the three characteristic qualities of the Cosmic Substance— sattva (stillness), *rajas* (action) and *tamas* (inertia). Both men and women should make efforts to understand each other better by accepting these differences, as well as taking into consideration the individual variations due to the fundamental constitution (*prakriti*) described in Ayurveda.

It is suggested that the education in companionship and sexuality should be imparted in an organised way to young people just as it was done in ancient India by the Ganikas (a special group of women who imparted this education). The book provides analysis and practical aspects of this education.

We have made a lot of progress in communication at technological level and our globe is like a village now. However at the level of intimacy between man and woman, we apply the ancient norms, which are not holistic and are based merely on need and convenience. The book emphasizes that in the modern times we need to change the way we look at a man-woman relationship. Just as we would not like to wear the clothes people wore a century ago, similarly, we should not use the old and redundant way of looking at a man-woman relationship as need-based alone.

Rituals and ceremonies are given to intensify the companionship and enhance sexual energy. There is a description of numerous aphrodisiacs to solve specific problems that hinder the flow of sexual energy and to enhance the sexual compatibility.